The THIN BOOK 2

BY JEANE EDDY WESTIN

CompCare®Publishers

2415 Annapolis Lane, Suite 140, Minneapolis, Minnesota 55441

Westin, Jeane Eddy.
  The thin book 2.

  Includes index.
    1. Reducing — Psychological aspects. I. Title.
II. Title: The thin book two.
RM222.2.W348   1984   613.2'5'019   84-14243
ISBN 0-89638-076-9 (pbk.)

Inquiries, orders, and catalog requests
should be addressed to
CompCare Publishers
2415 Annapolis Lane
Minneapolis, MN 55441
Call toll free 800/328-3330
(Minnesota residents 612/559-4800)

Book jacket design by Kristen McDougall

        5   6
       90 91

I thank my husband Gene, my family, my agent Jane Jordan Browne, and my editors for their untiring aid from conception to delivery. My deep appreciation also goes to those countless people who helped me with my own weight problem and with the formation of so many insights about recovering from a food compulsion.

All the material in this book is new, as my thinking about overweight has evolved over the years into the ideas you will read on these pages. Nevertheless, in a dozen years of writing about the problems of overweight, I have used some of the concepts and terms which appear in this book in other ways, particularly in my books *The Thin Book* and *Break Out of Your Fat Cell*.

Author's Introduction

Enough already! The arguments between all the diet experts are getting you nowhere.

The "know-thyselfers," the "magic diet group," and the "self-control specialists" each say they know best how to help you lose weight permanently. Some psychologists tell you to get in there, dig out all the mind-garbage, and you'll be whole. Great stuff, but you and I know hundreds of smart, self-aware fat people.

There are those who tout this week's low-cal, or high-protein, or low-carbohydrate, or no-fat, or no-cal diet plan — or this year's miracle diet ingredient — lecithin, sprouts, mega-vitamin therapy, or whatever. You've tried all these diets and more, so that's not the whole answer either.

Finally, there's what I call the-little-dieter-who-could advice: all you have to do is just keep trying and trying and you'll make it to Thinville. But again, this single-minded approach doesn't work.

None of this is worth a carrot stick alone. But what if you could blend the best from each, shake in the proper catalyst, and create a startlingly different plan? You'd have an exciting new, fat-attacking program. Do you agree with me on that so far? I hope so, because the main point of *The Thin Book 2* is that self-understanding (you'll learn why it's far better than self-awareness), plus dieting skills, plus determination will give you the kind of body and life you've always wanted, goals that have always seemed far beyond your grasp. But this will happen only if you know how to put these strategies into Action. Remember the word Action; it's a key.

Another key point of this book is that the choice to do anything in your life is yours, all yours. So what does that make you? It makes you the greatest asset in your own life; not those "experts" who haven't always got the answers, but you, because you *do* have the answers for yourself, if you can just uncover them. And because you are your greatest asset, it's about time you put your effort into encouraging yourself.

If you can give yourself everything, why haven't you?

The *mind experts* say it's because you lack self-esteem; the *diet experts* say it's because you haven't found the right diet; and the *you-can-do-it experts* say it's because you haven't tried hard enough yet. They're all right and they're all wrong.

Let's turn these old ideas upside-down. Let's assume that instead of having to acquire these attributes from outside experts, you already possess them. However, you also have blocks that often make you stumble when you call on your own strength. What if you had the power to kick these blocks aside? What if you knew what steps to take to get rid of the inner enemies that keep you from losing fat? Now, that changes everything, doesn't it? That makes each new day a challenge that doesn't get you down, but lifts you up. You can glory in such a day. It can be an adventure.

You already have everything you need. You just have to put it to work for you. Read that sentence again. Listen with your whole being to what it says about you. Isn't it exciting?

Say YES.

It's so easy to say YES to a new life, but so many overweights have forgotten how to say that little one-syllable word to themselves. So many of us, weighed down by failure after failure, become apathetic, even about our own lives. We wait to be motivated again. We have never learned, or we've forgotten if we once knew, that motivation is like a pump waiting to be primed. The way we prime it is to "get going." And how do we do that? We do it through what I call MindSteps.

MindSteps are principles of Action that you can turn into personal characteristics. They are so overlapping that to improve in only one means you improve in all the others too. The Twelve Action MindSteps you will learn in this book apply permanently to your weight problem and to your living problem; principles which will change your life's atmosphere forever.

The Twelve Action MindSteps

1. Develop a solid understanding of your unique worth.

2. Practice confidence every day.

3. Radiate warmth.

4. Learn what your fears are.

5. Acknowledge a burning desire to be thin and healthy.

6. Make your own sunlight.

7. Take charge of your life.

8. Do whatever needs to be done *now*.

9. Take weight loss in steps.

10. Reject rejection firmly and totally.

11. Don't fight inevitable change.

12. Play life to win.

There's a wonderful truth about The Twelve Action MindSteps: they don't wear out with use. Quite the contrary. They take you to greater depths and meanings with hard use — the harder the better. Your mind becomes clearer, your dieting skills strengthen, and your ability to drive ahead toughens. Can you imagine how this boosts your self-esteem? These twelve principles allow you to do what you want to do most.

That's a simple little thought, and yet it frightens overweight people more than it comforts. Isn't that so? Such a small thought and yet so terrifying. Why? Because we overweights feel helpless and hopeless. After all, we've been told so by experts (for example, the doctor who says, "If you can't follow orders, don't come back!"); and we've proved it to ourselves a thousand times. Until now the very thought of being in charge of our diets and our lives pushed us into tense, gloomy, and fearful attitudes. That is why, after every past diet success, we slipped back into the quagmire of overeating. It's true, isn't it? What we needed all the time was an attitude, a positive way to think about ourselves, and a way to reinforce those thoughts with Action.

The Thin Book 2 continues the process of help and hope started in *The Thin Book*, but with an additional Action message for people facing weight problems in our technological world. With all the books, articles, television specials, movies, tape cassettes, diet groups, and health information around, we overweights are probably the most self-aware people in the world. But self-awareness, so easy to acquire, is not self-understanding, which is quite a different set of learned mental attitudes. Therefore, the priority and focus of *The Thin Book 2* is self-understanding. In the end, you see, feel-good self-knowledge alone is useless, unless you put it into Action. In the following pages you'll find a course of daily Action — a plan for every day of the year, 365 days of Action leading you to your weight goal.

No one limits your success but you. If you want to be more, learn more, then do more. That's it. By adding *The Thin Book 2* to your daily self-help routine you will have to work a little harder for a while and spend a few more minutes each day, but there is a big pay-off. Most of you have jobs, professions, important duties which can be challenging and fun — life was meant to be fun, you know — but too much of your potential is trapped inside fat that condemns you to mere *existence.* Wouldn't you like to live thin and free of a need to overeat? Wouldn't you like a life that you could glory in? You and only you can make it happen. Turn on your mind. Learn The Twelve Action MindSteps. You and the MindSteps can be one; they can literally become you and you can become them. A few minutes a day with this book is all you need to lead you to life's winner's circle.

I was once where you are. I was young, loved, and reasonably intelligent but I overate in ways that made no sense to me. I thought I was crazy, or sick, or stupid. For thirty years, I was enormously fat and carried all the emotional baggage that goes with 272 highly visible pounds. Now, for fourteen years, I have been more than 100 pounds thinner and a hundred times happier with myself and my life.

But the good life didn't come to me because I needed it, or deserved it, or even because God wanted me to be thin. All those things are important. But I lost over 100 pounds and maintained that loss because I discovered something along the way: the absolute necessity of a daily mental, physical, and emotional/spiritual program, in addition to the diet I followed or the weight group I attended. A program of daily self-help to remind me where I had come from and where I wanted to go. Such day-by-day aids I have passed on in *The Thin Book* and *Break Out of Your Fat Cell* and supplement here in *The Thin Book 2.* Here I introduce The Twelve Action MindSteps which I discovered really make the difference between weight-losers and non-losers, weight-maintainers and non-maintainers.

Again, I am happy to be your supportive friend who helps make losing weight more positive and lasting than it ever was before. When you purchased this book you made an investment in yourself. Be proud of yourself for that.

You have the desire to control your overeating and change your life, or you wouldn't be reading these words right now. Isn't that right?

Say YES.

June, 1984
Sacramento, California

A Message from the Author to Twelve Step* Group Members

This book is a builder of self-esteem and self-reliance. It speaks to today's overeaters living on the near edge of the twenty-first century, who want to take responsibility for their own actions, accept the consequences of what they do, and take charge of their lives and health and emotional well-being. *The Thin Book 2* explains the difference between acting and only thinking about acting. It tells you to stop gearing up to lose weight, and encourages you to start doing it.

On the surface the "take charge of your life" philosophy of *The Thin Book 2* may seem to be at odds with AA's Twelve Step concepts as admission of powerlessness, surrender to a Higher Power, and humility. But is it? After closer examination, I think you'll find this book supplements those ideas in unique, practical ways.

Admitting that you are powerless as you do in the First Step does not mean quitting. It means that you stop denying you have a problem ("But I *like* to wear my navy blue raincoat in July!") and accept the need for change in your life. Such recognition is the foundation of all change.

Surrender in Twelve Step groups does not mean that you have no strength; it indicates a willingness to put aside defiance and open yourself to every source of help available.

Seventh Step humility ("humbly asked Him to remove our shortcomings") does not speak to a need for meekness in the overeater, which would seem to rule out a take-charge attitude. Humility in the Anonymous programs has far more subtle meanings. It's a recognition of personal worth, that you occupy a useful place in the scheme of things, and that you grant others their place, too. This idea, so beautifully rendered in CompCare

---

*The reference here is not to the author's Twelve Action MindSteps, but to the Twelve Steps of Alcoholics Anonymous (AA), also used by many other groups including Overeaters Anonymous (OA).

Publications' *Young Winners' Way*, makes the development of self-esteem an essential underpinning of humility.

The Twelve Steps of Overeaters Anonymous actually are the greatest calls to Action ever written. Nowhere do they say to surrender your problem with food to your Higher Power and then roll over and wait for the pounds to disappear. They say to admit, believe, decide, search, be fearless, be entirely ready, and to practice these principles in all your affairs. They add up to Action.

This book talks about the power of your mind to choose your own LifeWay, an idea that is compatible with the spiritual ideals of Anonymous groups. Indeed, free will is an important tenet of most of the world's religions. It means simply that when you ask for help, your Higher Power gives you choices, but *you* have to choose and follow through. The ultimate responsibility for change lies with you, doesn't it?

This book is intended to help you and thousands like you make good daily choices. Although you are responsible for carrying out a successful program, you are not alone. You have the Twelve Steps, your sponsor, your fellowship, wonderful literature, and, above all, your Higher Power. And now you have *The Thin Book 2*. Take the help you discover in these pages and get into Action today.

Please note: For maximum benefit *The Thin Book 2* is structured to be read to yourself, *out loud.*

My task . . . is to make you hear, to make you feel — and above all, to make you see. That is all, and it is everything.

Joseph Conrad

The Shape of Things to Come

*Enough, if something from our hands have power
To live, and act, and serve the future hour . . .*
William Wordsworth

A new year stretches ahead for you and you have the power in your hands to make a fresh beginning today. This is the day you're going to begin looking and feeling like a thinner winner; the day you're going to make the word "Action" the biggest word in your vocabulary. Why? Because you have made a YES decision about yourself, for today and all your future days.

But don't stop at decision-making. Don't even slow down. You can't live with good intentions only; decision without Action is like living in a house with no windows. Open your house to the light by putting your decision into Action. Take an Action step right now. Take the obvious one. Decide on a diet plan that will help you lose weight healthfully. Isn't that the logical first step? Then read the Twelve Action MindSteps once, and once again. Later you'll examine them one at a time, learn about each one of them in turn, and discover how beautifully they fit into your life. But today just become familiar with the sound of them in your head. Try them on. Believe me, they'll fit you like a glove. They were made for you!

What have you done right today? You've started the process of *becoming* these principles, of making Action a part of your daily life.

Today's Action Plan: Right where I am, from whatever weight, from whatever point of despair, I will make a strong positive start on my future.

Repeat and Repeat and Repeat

Repeat — iterate, reiterate, reproduce, echo, re-echo, drum, hammer, redouble, begin again, resume, return to.

Roget's Thesaurus

Repetition is the mother's milk of fat-free living. Repeating an Action makes it part of you, whether it's habitually choosing a healthful, weight-losing meal, or reinforcing a life-changing decision day after day. The more you repeat an Action, the more you make it all yours. Isn't that right?

But it has to be *effective* repetition, not distracted mindless sing-song. That means you must read it, write it, speak it, listen to it, then take Action and do it. It means that you have to repeat a positive Action until it dances in your head. That's vital, don't you agree?

What do great athletes do? They practice, they train, and they review the basics of their sport over and over again.

Repetition is a major ingredient of success. "Oh, that's boring," you say. "I've done all that. I know it. I haven't forgotten." But you have forgotten. Whatever it is that you're not doing right now, today, you're missing the benefit of its reinforcement, which is the entire reason for repeating an action in the first place.

What have you done right today? You have read the second page of this book. Read it again. Good! You practiced repetition. You just put yourself in training to become a winner.

Today's Action Plan: With every breath I take, I repeat the idea that the healthful life is worth reinforcing.

Your Unique Worth

When the fight begins within himself,
a man's worth something.

Robert Browning

The first Action MindStep says: **Develop a solid consciousness of your unique worth.** What does that mean? You can answer that question for yourself.

Some people project an unmistakable stamp of self-worth as soon as they enter a room. Their presence becomes a powerful force in the room. They reflect a sense of unique individuality that is beyond physical beauty or even good grooming. Their appearance is memorable, isn't it? You won't forget them. In fact, the memory of their impact can even haunt you. "What have they got that I haven't?" you ask. The answer is self-pride, not the overweening kind, but the honest pride that comes from capitalizing on their own potential — with a capital C.

You're cheating yourself if you don't believe in your unique worth. You're living life at a lower level than you deserve. Convince yourself that you're worth your greatest effort and you won't have to try to convince other people. They'll know it. They'll see it. They'll feel it.

What have you done right today? You have accepted the worthiness of your own best effort. Today you are convinced you have a right to a thinner, healthier body.

Today's Action Plan: When I walk through a door, I will radiate the unmistakable look of my unique worth. I will be a presence.

The Ingredients of Friendship

A friend is one to whom you may pour out all the contents of your heart, chaff and grain together, knowing that the gentlest of hands will take and sift it, keep what is worth keeping and with a breath of kindness blow the rest away.

Arabian Proverb

Wouldn't you like to have such a friend? Wouldn't you like to be such a friend to yourself? You would never allow anyone to treat you as hatefully as you sometimes have treated yourself. Isn't that right?

There are six qualities we expect from friends. We want them to *keep our confidences,* and share their *loyalty, warmth, affection, supportiveness,* and *sense of humor.* Is this what you bring to your best friend — yourself? Think about it for a minute. Do you stand up for yourself, and never, never show contempt for yourself in public? Do you deal gently with, and keep a sense of humor about, your foibles, "and with a breath of kindness, blow the rest away?"

You need your own friendship. It is absolutely impossible to live happily and healthfully without it. It comes down to this: you must become an expert in caring for your own precious life. At last you must give to yourself the quality of friendship you have been showering on others. Don't you agree?

What have you done right today? You have extended the gentle hand of friendship to the only person who can give you the winning thin life you desire.

Today's Action Plan: I will be a loving friend to myself. My friendship will have nothing whatever to do with what my weight is, but with what my need is.

4

Practicing Confidence

In quietness and in confidence shall be your strength.
Isaiah 30:15

The second Action MindStep says: **Practice confidence every day.** "How can I be confident," you ask, "when I'm a failure?" First, you're not a failure, and second, don't misunderstand this MindStep. It doesn't say *be* confident, it says *practice* confidence. There's a difference, isn't there?

"I'll be confident *after* I've lost weight," you say. "How can I have confidence before I've done it?"

It would be silly to advise anyone to walk out there in the world and be confident. That's like telling stutterers to just stop stuttering and they'll speak better. But practicing confidence is considerably easier to do, and gives the same results. Every day as you read and think about the Twelve Action MindSteps, you gain skill in the practice of confidence. Remember, people will be moved by your belief in yourself, by the conviction you display, and they will reflect back to you the confidence they see. What will they see? They will see that you have made a YES decision and have put it into Action. You can believe that, can't you?

What have you done right today? You have seen that each Action MindStep overlaps the others. Because you have faith in you unique worth, you have begun to radiate confidence.

Today's Action Plan: I will move in the world as if I'm an expert on myself. I will practice confidence until the act of practice becomes the essential me.

Eliminate the Negative

You gotta accentuate the positive,
eliminate the negative.

Johnny Mercer

Are you holding back from your weight goal because it might threaten someone? Do you feel your weight makes you a safer, less competitive friend, relative, mate, or lover, and that accounts for your popularity? You can't afford that kind of popularity. If you are delaying your own goals for someone else's sake, then somewhere you got the idea that success depends on acceptance by others, even negative people. This is a clear sign that you don't accept yourself. If your self-acceptance depends totally on pleasing others, you are riding a no-win horse.

Are you trying to get everyone to like you, even people who are a negative force in your life? We all love approval, but if you've drifted into seeking it from someone who doesn't support your living and weight goals, you're in a heap of trouble. But there's a way out.

Accentuate friendships with the positive people in your life. Limit those from whom you need approval to these positive people. That makes sense, doesn't it?

What have you done right today? You made a first step toward becoming your own person. You aren't demanding more approval than the world will give. You are no longer willing to live in the shadow of someone else's ego.

Today's Action Plan: I will not weaken my Action MindSteps in a vain attempt to gain recognition and approval. I will not be defeated before I have begun to fight.

Become an Expert in Caring

The only power which can resist the power of fear is the power of love.

Alan Paton

The third Action MindStep says: **Radiate warmth.**
Become an expert in caring. "Oh sure," you say, "another smarmy platitude that I've been hearing since my mother told me to say nothing about anyone if it wasn't nice." Is that what you think caring is? Not quite. (Although Mom had a point.)

The reason you should show care for others is this: we are so afraid others won't like us that our fear is often misinterpreted as icy reserve. How you feel about yourself is what you project to other people. If you project warmth and caring (even if you have to make a real effort at first), others will see you as that kind of person and mirror their view in the way they respond to you. You're beginning to see now, aren't you?

By radiating warmth and caring, you are saying to the world that you have a reservoir of love, that you have made a YES decision about yourself that you are going to share with others.

Don't forget that the people in your life will believe what you do, not what you say. You can understand how that could be so, can't you?

What have you done right today? Action is going to work for you in ways that all the other magic methods never did. You have begun to understand that each Action MindStep is part of a total system that will take you stride-by-stride down the winning road in life.

Today's Action Plan: I will discover for myself the changes that warmth and caring will bring into my life. I will overpower my fear of the first person I meet — with love.

Don't Ask Yourself the Wrong Questions

*No question is so difficult to answer as that to which
the answer is obvious.*

George Bernard Shaw

"Why can't I do anything right?" "What's wrong with
me?" Some overeaters seem to wallow in destructive self-
criticism, to glory in hopelessness and self-belittling and
put-downs. Most of the time these are silent questions,
creating a continuing monologue. You know that kind of
talk, don't you?

Self-questioning can be positive, if it's done to discover
where you went wrong and how to avoid that mistake in
the future. But when it's a destructive argument to berate
yourself, forget it. If you keep on asking, "What's wrong
with me?," soon you will find yourself convinced that
you are indeed worthless. You'll begin to believe that
everything you do is wrong, that you will fail. And then
you *will* fail.

Send your mind positive questions. Ask, "What did I
do right?" and "How could I do even better?"

You need an inner voice that's a friend, not an enemy;
that's smart, positive, and true. You do need that, don't
you?

What have you done right today? You have learned
why you should read the question "What have you done
right today?" out loud, every day. You can see why this
question is repeated daily on these pages. You realize the
importance of asking yourself "right" questions so you
will get "right" answers.

Today's Action Plan: I will ask "What is good about
me?" I will not abuse myself, but be a loving friend.

The Greatest De-motivator

We have nothing to fear but fear itself.
Franklin D. Roosevelt

The fourth Action MindStep says: **Learn what your fears are.** If you know your fears, they can't jump out and take you unaware. Essentially, most of us are afraid of one thing, failure. Oh, we call it by many other names, but behind them all lurks the fear of lost prestige — failure. That's it. Take the time to examine your fears honestly, one by one. Now, don't you agree?

You're not really afraid of others, of things that go bump in the night, or dark places. You're mostly afraid of being inadequate — a failure. How many times have you given up on yourself as a diet failure? How many?

Don't reject yourself. It always triggers fear. You express fear as anxiety, and anxiety mimics hunger. You know the rest . . . .

It's a good thing to take a daily inventory of your fears because fear — the biggest de-motivator of all — stops you cold. Frankly, most people can't remember what they were afraid of last week. Fear is a habit, and has little to do with reality.

From this day on, replace fear with what you desire from life. Think about that healthful thin body you want so desperately, and this positive image will motivate you, push you forward. Make a strong start. You'd like to do that, wouldn't you?

What have you done right today? You've taken the first small step toward ridding your life of its impossible load of fear. You are a help, not a burden, to yourself.

Today's Action Plan: I will overcome fear by denying it the power to make me overeat. I will remember that fear is only an acronym for False Evidence Appearing Real.

The Simple Lesson We Haven't Learned

The future starts today, not tomorrow.
                                        Pope John Paul II

"I'll think about that tomorrow," said Scarlett O'Hara in the last scene of *Gone With The Wind.* That may be all right for Miss Scarlett in her scheme to get Rhett Butler back, but for the rest of us it's a loser's philosophy.

Don't hedge your commitment to a new life by endless postponing. "I'll start a healthful, lifetime eating program tomorrow," you say, "or Monday, or New Year's Day."

You've said all these things before, haven't you?

Starting today — right now — commit yourself to diet success. Don't weaken your resolve to do the difficult things you must do with an I'll-give-it-a-try attitude. No ifs or buts. Don't excuse yourself from an all-out effort.

You get a bonus for your commitment. It's really exciting to know you're in charge, and that you will not deny yourself what you want from life. Defying procrastination is one good habit that guarantees success.

Remember, all habits are learnable, including this one. Make it one of yours. You'd like that, wouldn't you?

What have you done right today? You have committed yourself to a positive new way of thinking about the future. This is because you are tired of postponing happiness, and living on wishes and lies. You have accepted the simple idea that *today*, not tomorrow, is the beginning of the rest of your life.

Today's Action Plan: Right now I will replace the bad habit of procrastination with the good habit of working for what I want. I will start from where I am, as I am.

The Good Craving

desire: to wish or long for; crave
American Heritage Dictionary

The fifth Action MindStep says: .**Acknowledge a burning desire to be thin and healthy.** You have to provide the desire to succeed. Start with a want, a desire, a craving for a thin body. Nobody can be a winner without enormous desire, and the more you desire, the more you will help yourself do what it takes to lose weight. Not just general wanting — happiness, health, money — but focus on specific wants: 20 pounds, strong legs, dollars for a vacation. Make agreements with yourself: "If I do this, I'll get that." Don't work for nothing. That's smart, isn't it?

We overeaters like to keep our wants secret — even from ourselves. If we don't acknowledge how much we want to be thin, it won't hurt so much if we fail. Is hiding this desire for success the way to protect us from diet failure? No! Our wants power our drive to win. Rather than hide them, we should hold them out in front of us as we go and develop positive cravings for them. This is a good craving, a wonderful craving.

You know you have the capacity to crave. Don't fight it, use it. Use it wholeheartedly and it will ignite the fuse of your diet program. You believe that, don't you?

What have you done right today? You have learned to turn the liability of craving into an asset. You have begun to harness the power of wanting to the desire to succeed.

Today's Action Plan: I will acknowledge to myself and to others my burning desire to be thin and healthy. I will bring all my craving power to bear on my weight goal.

Begin Where You Are

*Don't let life discourage you; everyone who got where
he is had to begin where he was.*
Richard L. Evans

You want to lose weight and free the essential you that
lives inside a fleshy prison, but you're having trouble
starting. Your need is urgent, consuming, as it must be in
order to achieve success. But even desperately wanting to
lose weight doesn't tell you where to begin, does it?

Start any way, anywhere, and the pieces will fall into
place for you. When an overeater asked a recovered
alcoholic, "Give me the answer so that I can begin," he
responded, "Begin so you can get the answer."

Just as you are, you are complete. You are capable of
beginning just where you are. Believe that. Begin.

You don't even need to be enthusiastic. If you act
enthusiastic, you'll become enthusiastic. At first, you
might have to fake it, but then it will come. It will!

What have you done right today? You see that just by
starting you are a step closer to achieving. You understand that the time and place to begin are right now and
right here — and for all you're worth.

**Today's Action Plan: I will believe that the time to
start is now. I will begin from wherever I am to find my
answer on the other side of Action.**

I Am My Sunshine, My Only Sunshine

A man should learn to watch that gleam of light which flashes across his mind from within . . .
Ralph Waldo Emerson

The sixth Action MindStep says: **Make your own sunlight.** Don't wait for everyone else to feel good before you do. You're mistaken if you think this principle suggests you play little Miss Sunshine, tip-tapping your way around the Good Ship Lollipop. It doesn't mean that at all. It simply means that you take charge of your own happiness. That's clear so far, isn't it?

Why should your happiness depend on other people and events? Why should you be enthusiastic and full of joy only when everybody else is up? That takes the power out of your inner self and places it in the hands of other people.

Being happy is one habit you should cultivate. Work on the happiness habit. Your habits are your choices.

That's not very sympathetic, is it? But when you're unhappy, you don't need pity. You need to win. Winners are happy people who attract other winners. That's what you need. Sympathy never helped you lose one pound, did it?

What have you done right today? You have seen that happiness is a light that shines from the inside out. As with every Action MindStep, if you want it, do it.

Today's Action Plan: I will light my own way to happiness. I won't wait for others, but will get into Action myself.

LifeWay

Life is a mirror and will reflect back to the thinker what he thinks into it.

Ernest Holmes

"Lifestyle" popularly means a mode of life. You won't find that word in this book because it seems too frivolous, too transitory a word to describe your new life, a life based on the principles of Action embodied in the Twelve MindSteps. You do agree, don't you?

In this book you'll read the word LifeWay, representing your way of living free from excess food. It conveys a sense of permanence, not fad; of continuity, not fashion; of an anchor, not something you put on and take off easily.

When you select your right-eating plan, choose physical exercise, and adopt MindStep attitudes, these things *become* your LifeWay. They help you build new habits of success and sustain them. You move from simple self-awareness to Action oriented self-understanding. At last, you found a way to make sense out of your life!

Your LifeWay helps you develop a zest for success; former failures are now challenges, you are self-confident and victory-conscious. You acquire the kind of faith and optimism that sets winners apart from losers — you know you can succeed. That is the vision of your LifeWay, isn't it?

What have you done right today? You adopted the idea of your life encapsulated in one word, LifeWay. You know that great success is on its way.

Today's Action Plan: I will choose my own LifeWay. I will base it on a vision of victory.

The Most Important Day of Your Life

The world is for those who make their dreams come true.

Harold Gray

You're holding this book in your hands because you think it can help you lose weight and maintain it. This probably isn't the only "diet" book you've read, and maybe you're wondering, "Hey, where's the new diet?" All right, here it is: it's a magical diet, a mental diet that not only insures that you lose weight, but guarantees that you will live sunny-side up for the rest of your life. You're ready for that, aren't you?

Now read these words. Commit them to memory. And commit all your energy to the seventh Action MindStep (the most important of the twelve) which says: **take charge of your life.** If life is a feast, be the host, not the guest. There it is. That's all.

That doesn't mean that you should run around belligerently yelling, "I'm mad as hell and I'm not going to take it anymore!" That's angry self-pity thinly disguised as Action. Feeling sorry for yourself is the biggest loser's trap of all time. It kills everything in you that it takes to be a winner. Taking charge of your life means you'll have to do it by yourself and for yourself. Nobody can fix your life for you. You understand, don't you?

What have you done right today? You learned the most important Action MindStep of all. You are ready to take responsibility for yourself, which includes putting together your own living plan.

Today's Action Plan: I will take charge of my own life. At the feast of life, I will sit at the head of the table.

Yes, You Can

What goes around, comes around.
Contemporary saying

"Been down so long it looks like up to me," says the old one-liner. Not too funny when you feel this way, is it? When you're overweight in a thin-is-in society, it's easy to feel depressed, frustrated, humiliated, rejected, deprived, and punished, and that's just in the morning. Winners can't allow any such negative feelings to interfere with their goals. If so, goals become just wishes without fairy godmothers. Isn't that right?

There is a prescription for depression called the Negative question/Action answer. It works like this. If you catch yourself thinking or saying, "I can't lose ten pounds," you reply out loud, "Yes, I can!" Out loud now. You need to hear yourself taking charge of your weight problem.

And by the way, forget about the little voice inside you that whispers all too logically: "You've always failed before; you'll fail again." Nonsense! Such logic is for losers, not winners. You are not condemned to carry the past around on your shoulders forever.

A diet of negativity guarantees you'll fail; nourishing yourself with positive responses guarantees you'll win. Winners say YES to life. Makes a lot of sense, doesn't it?

What have you done right today? You have become a YES person. You have begun to see that the fight against fat may be as much in your head as on your plate.

Say YES.

Today's Action Plan: Very few people get to where I want to go, but I can be one of them. Yes, I can.

Living in the Now

Dost thou love life? Then do not squander time, for that's the stuff life is made of.
Benjamin Franklin

The eighth Action MindStep says: **Do whatever has to be done now.** It will never be today again, so use today to take Action that will change your life.

The purpose of this book is to inspire you to change, so you can become a winner. True, there is stress in any diet, job, or social change. But you are stressed much more from changes that are thrust on you than from your own take-charge changes. That's the way it's always been, hasn't it?

Refusal to change, to grow, to meet challenges, cuts the pattern of defeat deep into your life. Remember this: You aren't judged by how often you fail, but by how many times you win. Here's the important part: you'll win in direct proportion to how many times you can fail but keep on beginning again.

Think about the people you admire most. It's their fighting spirit, their ability to seize the moment and get on with the job that attracts you, isn't it?

What have you done right today? First, you are more able to get to work on today's task. Second, you have learned that beginning again and again is the stuff each day is made of. And you have it in you to do it.

Today's Action Plan: I will get on with my life's work. I will use each minute because it will never come again.

The Word that You Forgot

Everything has been said before, but since nobody listens we have to keep going back and beginning all over again.

André Gide

Say YES. You've heard it before, and you'll hear it again. Is the word "yes" hard for you to say to yourself? Say it again, YES. There you go!

We overweights are often such people-pleasers. We run around looking for ways to say "yes" to other people so they'll like us, maybe even forget we're fat. Oh, we're good at pleasing other people. Aren't we?

But when it comes to pleasing you, what do you say? "No!" It was the first word your parents taught you. "No, no, no!" They knew that you'd hurt yourself if you didn't learn to avoid fire, and stairs, and broken glass. But they didn't want you to keep saying "no" to yourself, to your dreams, and to your desires, for the rest of your life.

You've heard it all before. You've been preached at so often that you've learned to turn a deaf ear. This time you should pay attention as if your life — the good life — depends on it. It does. Now say YES. Say YES to an eating plan that will help you take off your excess weight, and keep it off. You were listening this time, weren't you?

What have you done right today? You have learned to work positively with yourself. When there is more yes than no in your life, you will wake each morning to an exciting day that you'll look forward to. Say YES, and mean it. Are you listening?

Today's Action Plan: I will listen to whatever I have to for as long as it takes me to learn it. I will take no out of my life and put YES in.

Step by Step

*If you have no idea where you want to go, it makes
little difference how fast you travel.*

Italian Proverb

The ninth Action MindStep is: **Take weight loss in steps.**
If you've never been at your natural weight, don't target
it for next month. Always aim for a weight goal that
excites you, but doesn't frighten you. Then when you
reach that goal, start the process all over again until you
reach your ultimate goal. That puts you in charge,
doesn't it?

Setting goals is easy for most overeaters. We're such
all-or-nothing people that, in the first wave of enthusiasm, we decide to lose all our excess weight now. We're
fine until we run into our first problems. Then we
stumble, depression sets in, and we overeat. This is a
scene most of us have enacted again and again.

Who created the problems? You did, by setting unrealistic goals. There are numbers on your scale that are
natural resting points. You know them because they are
weights that you have probably maintained for a time.
When setting your weight loss goals, aim for the first
familiar resting point. Stop there and say, "Well done."
Then start again. If you try to rush on by, you'll stumble
every time. Isn't that right?

What have you done right today? You have decided
to set reasonable priorities, well thought out in advance.
You are thrilled by your first weight goal.

**Today's Action Plan: I will set my next goal. I will
write it down and commit myself to reaching it.**

Choosing Your Diet

Unfortunately, people ask more of car salesmen than they do about new diets. Some of the fads that have been promoted are outrageous . . . .

Dr. Peter Wood

Most weight control plans provide a meal-by-meal listing of what to eat for a specified period. With the menus are usually two other lists: one list of foods you can eat in unlimited quantities, another list of foods you should avoid totally. This kind of diet may be one way to get started, but as soon as possible you should choose your own right-eating plan. You'd like to do that, wouldn't you?

You need a new definition of diet. Think of it not as something to "go on" so you can eventually "go off" it, but as the way you want to live with food now and forever, an integral part of your LifeWay.

The best diet plan is one that follows general nutritional guidelines — for example, a diet which calls for a mixture of protein, unsaturated fat, and carbohydrates.

Your right-eating plan should be high in natural fiber, with plenty of grains, fruits, and vegetables; and it should be low in salt, sugar and saturated fats. Red meats and dairy products, if allowed, should be used in moderation. This is a diet for energy, health, and weight control. That's what you want, isn't it?

What have you done right today? You decided to choose your right-eating plan, using these guidelines for food selection.

Today's Action Plan: I will choose a diet I can live with for a lifetime. I will make it the first part of my three-part LifeWay.

Rejection

*If fifty million people say a foolish thing it is still a
foolish thing.*

Anatole France

The tenth Action MindStep says: **Reject rejection firmly
and totally.** How much do you depend on the opinion of
others? When your mate or a friend disapproves of your
new resolve, saying, "Ugh, another diet. I suppose that
means we won't get any decent meals around here."
What do you do? Do you back off from your goals
rather than risk losing that person? That's a mistake, one
of the biggest. Don't blame yourself too much if you
have been marching to someone else's drum beat. All
your life, you've understood that you're nobody 'til
somebody loves you. That's what you've heard, isn't it?

If people reject you because they don't like your goals,
reject their rejection, completely. What they're really
objecting to is that you have become your own new
"center of gravity." They are uncomfortable with your
emerging independence; they see that you are no longer
dependent on their awareness, but are inner-directed
toward your own.

It's true, you may be lonely for a time; you may even
miss looking up to someone for acceptance. That's the
price you pay for finally being able to take charge of
your life. You can't have it both ways; you must choose.
You're too old for a baby-sitter anyway, aren't you?

What have you done right today? You have discovered how the trap of dependence is built, so you can
work your way out of it. You have gladly traded
dependence for independence.

**Today's Action Plan: I will reject rejection. I will be a
self-directed person.**

Your Full Life

Life can be so full, if you use it.
Laura Z. Hobson

One of the dictionary definitions of the word "use" is to consume. When applied to life, that's an interesting concept for overeaters. Instead of excess food, life itself is what we should be consuming, or devouring. It may be that we overeaters choose the wrong approach. Instead of thinking of life using (devouring) us, let's think of using life to its absolute fullest. You can change your thinking, can't you?

There's a contemporary axiom which is applied to everything except living: "use it or lose it." How apt, don't you think? If you don't approach life with a fresh zest every day, you can lose it a day at a time. Sad, time is so precious.

Plan your time. If you don't know how, start with this simple, effective system: set aside a few minutes every morning (same time, same place, to make it a firm habit) and actually write down the Action MindStep you're going to concentrate on for the rest of the day. Working on MindSteps can supplement other programs — spiritual or physical — which are aimed at achieving your weight goals. Go ahead, plan each day so you can live life to the brim. You're going to do that, aren't you?

What have you done right today? You have discovered a new life-saving idea, to use life instead of allowing it to use you. You have found a daily system of using your precious time.

Today's Action Plan: I will plan my time today. I will make full use of every minute.

Change — the Challenge

*Risk is essential. There is no growth or inspiration in
staying within what is safe and comfortable.*
Alex Noble

The eleventh Action MindStep says: **Don't fight inevitable change.** Make change work for you. You can't stay
the same. Changes come in your life, no matter what
you do to stop them. Since change is inevitable, the best
changes will be those you control. Look back at the
changes in your life thus far, those forced on you, and
those you chose. Which ones made you feel more in
charge of your own destiny? Look back right now, won't
you?

In the pages of this book, you will be asked many
times to look into your inner self, to unfold and find in
yourself the knowledge you will need to march ahead to
a healthier, happier, winning life. You will be taking a
journey through a mindscape of your thoughts, feelings,
memories, urges — the mental and emotional essence
that is uniquely you. This trip inside your mind will help
you discover for yourself the unconscious negative motivations that make you use food in ways you do. That
will be some trip, won't it?

What have you done right today? You have accepted
that change is a part of life's system. And, you have
decided that, whenever possible, you will make your
own choices. Take your place with the winners.

**Today's Action Plan: I will control change when I can,
so that from now on I will be the driver, not the
passenger. I will become as familiar with my own
mindscape as I am with the picture on my wall.**

Courage, Friend

Keep on keeping on.
Alcoholics Anonymous saying

Most likely you picked up this book hoping to discover something of value. Oh yes, you have hope, all right. Sometimes it's such a flickering little flame that it seems ready to burn out, but somehow it doesn't. You go on. Do you know why you go on as you do? Because you have courage. That's what hope is, the courage to go on, and then to go on again, in the face of the most mind-numbing defeat. Don't be modest. That's true, isn't it?

Picking up this book and reading it, thinking about it, and putting its ideas into Action, illustrates something about your kind of bravery. You have the courage it takes to live with a food problem in our thin-is-best culture, and keep that tiny pilot light of hope glowing.

This book isn't concerned with fantasy heroes nor bemedaled vanquishers, but rather with people who fall down and get up, fight a problem and whip it. This book is about *continuing,* the character trait that will lead you to lifelong triumphs. Think about that today, won't you?

What have you done right today? You have learned something positive about yourself, that the tiny flame of hope is really like a pilot light ready to burst into full blaze with the slightest encouragement. Your reading these lines shows you have kept the flame alive. That's Courage, my friend.

Today's Action Plan: I will recognize that my average life is made above average by the hope I keep alive. I will put my courage into Action and follow my eating plan.

The Weight of the Evidence

There is always an enormous temptation in all of life to diddle around . . . it is so self-conscious, so apparently moral, simply to step aside from the gaps where the creeks and winds pour down, saying, I never merited this grace . . . and then to sulk along the rest of your days on the edge of rage. I won't have it.

Annie Dillard

The twelfth and last of the Action MindSteps says: **Play life to win.** People are apt to be apathetic, even about their own welfare. Beyond their immediate satisfactions, they are satisfied just to get by. Well, that's not good enough for you! You have wants. You want a thinner body. You want to achieve more, to be more successful. But above all, you want some peace of mind, a way out of the pit of overeating, don't you?

Life's winners don't get to be winners because they "diddle around." They set goals and do what has to be done to achieve them. Winners don't live by the grazing principle, a little here, a little there, with no end in mind. They make plans and head straight for their goals. By the time they reach them, they have learned to love themselves enough to believe they deserve what they've worked so hard for. You can believe that, can't you?

What have you done right today? You have decided that life is too short to wander around with no goal in mind. You know that your next goal and your good eating plan will get you to where you want to go. You believe that you deserve what you get.

Today's Action Plan: I will not fool around in this life waiting to be rescued. Failure — I won't have it!

The Twelve Action MindSteps

Nothing is impossible to the man who can will, and then do; this is the only law of success.
Honoré Mirabeau

Do more than just read the Twelve Action MindSteps. Study them, memorize them, let the ideas sink in. In this book, we'll go back to them again and again. It takes a lot of repeating to undo years of overeating. Take time to know the MindSteps, will you?

Expect to have a few rough days. Your life won't turn around dramatically in twenty-four hours, but it's surprising how fast you *do* begin to feel better about yourself. Just don't forget while you're having one of those bad days, that if you'll keep on working, keep on learning, keep on doing, the rough period will pass and the good days will come. This works every time.

Don't make it grim. Schedule non-food rewards when you've earned them. (Never reward yourself with anything when you haven't earned it — we overweights have already done too much of that.) And don't miss taking your rewards. Don't cheat yourself out of some puritan sense of self-punishment. Rewards help you to maintain a strong drive toward your goal. That's perfectly obvious, isn't it?

What have you done right today? You have learned that winners have to work hard to assimilate the Twelve Action MindSteps. When you deserve it, give yourself a positive non-food reward, like recreation, a new gadget, or anything you really want. Keep your motivation and will to win high; take the rewards you earn.

Today's Action Plan: I will take one Action step at a time, again and again. My life will be beautiful.

Self-responsible Living

*There is no dependence that can be sure
but a dependence on one's self.*

John Gay

You've tried the rest, now why not try your best? You've found any number of trendy diet and fitness books which provided reducing diets and fitness regimens all laid out for you. This book asks you to discover your own personal LifeWay, and that includes managing your own nutrition and exercise programs. You can do that, can't you?

Many weight-control programs failed simply because they didn't fit you as an individual. They demanded too many capricious compromises with the way you want to live. The program was master and you were the servant.

No single weight-losing or exercise regimen is exactly right for anybody. There are many good ones, but they are only foundations on which to build your own way of eating and energizing. Learning how to take care of your body and your life is an essential process of independence. No one can hand you a ready-made solution; you must mold your own.

Following your own plan, there is no competition, no other schedule for success. And there's no reason to delay because you fear you won't measure up to others. Repeat the phrase, "my own way." Doesn't it have the ring of freedom?

What have you done right today? You decided to discover your own path to physical and mental fitness. You believed that you must become the primary expert on your own life.

Today's Action Plan: I will take responsibility for my own life plan. I will follow my personalized schedule to independence.

The "If" that Stands Between

Let no one or anything stand between you and the difficult task, let nothing deny you this rich chance to gain strength by adversity, confidence by mastery, success by deserving it. Do it better each time. Do it better than anyone else can do it. I know this sounds old-fashioned. It is, but it has built the world.

Harlow H. Curtice

Are you saying, "If I were younger — " or "If I weighed less — " or "If I were smarter — " I'd try the Twelve Action MindSteps. Only an "if" stands between you and fulfillment. Only an "if" keeps you from the most exciting turning point in your life. What are you going to do about"if"?

Whether you just started a weight-control program or you've been at it for years, determine today that you will make this book pay off for you.

Early morning is the best time to absorb the day's message. Underline words or phrases that are important to you. Jot them on a slip of paper. Repeat them to yourself

during the day. Use what you learn right away to help you live better.

What is your present state of mind? Are you paying complete attention? Concentrate, absorb, and think while you read. Firmly plant each day's thoughts in your memory.

You'll do that, won't you? Say YES, not IF.

What have you done right today? You let this book encourage you to sell yourself to yourself. You learned to keep "if" from getting between you and fulfillment.

Today's Action Plan: I will absorb each day's message. I will use it to help me when an "if" gets in my way.

The Good Witch of Oz

*The Wicked Witch of the West said, "I could make her
my slave, for she does not know how to use
her power."*

L. Frank Baum

You have the power to rescue yourself. (That's what the
Good Witch of the South told Dorothy in *The Wizard of
Oz*, and that's what this book tells you.) Deep in your
inner self, your word is the supreme law. In recent years,
it has become psychologically popular to blame others
for our problems. "That's just another rotten thing my
mother did to me," or, "If I had married the right man
(woman), I wouldn't need to overeat." We've all looked
for someone or something to blame for our extra
pounds, haven't we?

The power is right there inside you, the power to do
as you want to do; to cooperate with yourself in a new
way to eat; to build a new LifeWay. If you don't possess
this power over yourself, then who does? Who is
responsible for your ability to think, move, and work?
Nobody else pulls the strings when you function. You
tell yourself to do all of these things, and then you do
them.

The greatest endeavor of your life is the discovery of
the infinite mind power that you can use. Believe that,
will you?

What have you done right today? You uncovered the
good and the powerful in you. You pictured yourself as
you have always wanted to be: a winner.

**Today's Action Plan: I won't settle for anything less
than to learn how to use my own power. When I need
strength, I will look to the limitless power of my mind.**

Are You Willing?

The alcoholic has to be in such pain that he is willing to do anything, even get well!
Alcoholics Anonymous saying

Like alcoholism, overeating can be a terrible addiction — with one difference. The overeater cannot completely give up eating, but must continue to "feed the habit" at least three times a day. While the alcoholic can be rid of alcohol, and the drug addict can be free of damaging chemical substances, the overeater must make a life companion of food. There must be another way out of the morass of food-dependence, mustn't there?

The way out is to change your thinking, change those ingrained habits. It will take daily vigilance. Know that, if you want to overeat, no amount of wishing, will power, tears or tantrums, can make you give up your inner want. To change your habit, you must change the want.

You certainly don't want the bloat, nausea, and sugar-shakes that go with overeating. What if you truly learned to dislike overeating, to hate it? Getting rid of something you hate is entirely different from giving up something you like. You see the difference, don't you?

What have you done right today? You saw that you are your own jailer. You learned that you are "getting rid" of a terrible food addiction, not "giving up" anything good.

Today's Action Plan: I want to leave overeating behind. I am so sick and tired of pain that I'm willing to get well, no matter what it takes.

The Supreme Excitement

There are plenty of alibis for failure; success doesn't need them.

Anonymous

One excitement for every overeater is supreme: the excitement and deep satisfaction of reaching a weight goal, and then going on to a new one. You finally understand that weight loss is a continuing process, you never cease building new attitudes and using the inner power you have discovered. You are beginning to understand that knowing what you think and why you think that way isn't enough, you must put this knowledge into Action. You can feel this happening, can't you?

You have learned the value of time. If you postpone today, you lose it. Now is all you have. No matter how difficult your problem, no matter how long you've lived with it, you have begun to think about how to be good to yourself today. It's certainly time for that — past time!

You want something more from life than you've had, and you know what it is. Every day you live, every move you make, is a way of getting a thinner body and a healthier attitude. You start with this goal each day, and then you swing into Action, don't you? Say YES.

What have you done right today? You looked back over the month of January, and you can see that your life is beginning to change. You learned more about your own mindscape than you ever knew before.

Today's Action Plan: I will put my positive new attitudes into Action. I will live today as if it were all there was to life.

Beginning

The beginning is half of every action.
                                              Greek proverb

Today is a new opportunity for you. To be successful, some overeaters begin anew every day. They need strong motivation to put each day on a positive path, so they perform a ritual of beginning. To reinforce their goal the ritual could be an inspirational reading, a supportive telephone call to another overeater, or prayer. Develop your own ritual for an Action day. Each morning, seek a balance between what the world demands, and what you must do for yourself. Don't give all your time and energy to the "busy work" of living. You can do that, can't you?

Make a good beginning. If you see difficulties ahead, try to eliminate or work around them. Plan to take every opportunity to achieve your personal goals.

Motivating yourself to do what you already know you should do is the main problem, always. What do you want to accomplish today? You can make anything happen. The choice is always yours, because you aren't now and never were helpless. If you threw away most of the mental power you've used so far, you would still have more than you could ever use. To strengthen it, use it. Positive mental attitudes are like muscle; the more you exercise them, the stronger they become. These skills never wear out. That's a wonderful truth, isn't it?

What have you done right today? You developed a positive ritual for starting each day. You are taking charge; you are setting goals. Now, you have the idea!

Today's Action Plan: I will make a good beginning. I will exercise my positive mental muscles.

Establish Routine

*You will never be the person you can be if pressure,
tension and discipline are taken out of your life.*
                                            Dr. James G. Bilkey

Overeaters usually lack discipline. Of course, there are
some who lead fairly organized lives when they aren't
dealing with food, but they are a minority. Continuous
snacking and over-emphasis on food interrupt daily life
so it's difficult to maintain schedules. Are you nodding
yes so far?

Setting a time for doing what you want to accomplish
is beneficial. Repeating an activity at the same time every
day helps to make the activity — exercise, for example
— habitual.

Give priorities to the things you want to get done.
Your highest priorities should include meal planning for
right-eating and all the shopping and preparation that
goes with it. Other high priorities are exercise, today's
Action plan, and your work and family. All other
activities come later.

Now that you've given structure to your day, the
schedule won't mean much unless you follow it. Planning isn't Action. Following your routine today, tomorrow and afterwards — that's Action. Do it, won't you?

What have you done right today? You set time and
priorities for the things you want to accomplish. Now
that you have a plan, you will follow it.

**Today's Action Plan: I will put my LifeWay priorities
first. I will create routines of healthy, happy new habits.**

Are You a List-maker?

*Any plan that depends upon luck to succeed
isn't a plan; it's a gamble.*

Anonymous

Don't just read this book, use it! When you read an
interesting idea, write it down. List it with the things you
want to accomplish today. Successful people are structured people. They don't rely on memory or luck to
remind them of what they want to do. They make lists.
Be a list-maker. Will you say YES?

First make a list of what you want to do today. But
next, and most important, do the tasks. Making the list
is not Action. *Doing* is the key to your new thin life.
Before you go to bed at night, check off your list every
item you accomplished or draw a heavy line through it.
Now that's a satisfying feeling.

When you have the list habit, you feel more dynamic
and goal-oriented. You're actually ahead of non-list-
makers because you don't have to waste time wondering
what it was you wanted to do with your day.

Lists seem to hatch new lists. Some lists are more
important and become permanent. Tack those up where
you can refer to them often. Other lists are quickly
accomplished — Today's Action Plan at the bottom of
every page is one of these — and give way to a new list
every day. Lists are tools. You can use them creatively,
can't you?

What have you done right today? You recognized that
lists help you organize your day, which helps forestall
overeating from frustration. Get out your paper and
pencil!

Today's Action Plan: I will list the things I want to
accomplish. I will organize my day to exclude overeating.

Is Overeating a Disease?

*disease: to interrupt or impair any or all the natural
and regular functions of an organ of a living body*
            Webster's Unabridged Dictionary

Does habitual overeating impair the regular or natural
functions of your body in any way? Let's see. Have you
ever felt logy, hung over from too much sugar, tired,
dizzy, generally debilitated? If you have, what would
you call your overeating?

For the sake of argument, let's say that you really feel
your general health is good. Besides, you can't buy the
idea of overeating as a disease. Sounds too radical to
you.

Let's look at the word disease another way: dis-ease —
to make uneasy, to distress. That definition hits home,
doesn't it?

Overeating is a disease of living, and its symptom is
fat. Food became a drug to protect you from a negative
personal view of life where you saw yourself always
losing, always at the mercy of people and situations.

The disease of excess hunger is curable. You simply
have to form a winning view of the world and your
place in it. The Twelve Action MindSteps, coupled with
right-eating
and body rebuilding exercise, are the answer. Come
on, begin your recovery, won't you?

What have you done right today? You were willing to
accept a new concept. You no longer reject any idea or
method that can help you become a thinner winner.

**Today's Action Plan: I will be grateful that I can
recover from my "disease." I will take the MindSteps as
prescribed.**

Oh, What Good Confusion

oxymoron: a paradoxical conjunction of terms
American Heritage Dictionary

What is good confusion? Isn't confusion of any kind supposed to be bad for us? Generally, yes, but in the context of this book, no. When you seek self-understanding, your mind may indulge in confusion to protect itself from change. If you are confused, that's acceptable. Don't question it. Accept confusion as another step toward self-understanding. You can go along with that idea, can't you?

Do you ever feel there is another person inside you, a fabulous personality, a special someone just under the surface, more alive than the self you know so well? You, but with a lot more to you?

Are you ready to unchain that other part of you, the real, more powerful you? If your answer is YES, expect confusion, because confusion reflects the conflict between what your outer self denies, and what your inner self knows. Gradually, as you grow in self-understanding, you will literally pull yourself inside out. Don't expect the process to come easily. The more we understand, the more we know there is to understand. It's a rebirth process. Do you believe it?

What have you done right today? You realized that confusion is part of your learning process. You have caught a glimpse of the fabulous reality within you.

Today's Action Plan: Step by step I will gain understanding. I will cultivate an inquiring attitude so I can release my confident inner self.

Where the Answer Lies

Be a lamp unto your own feet,
do not seek outside yourself.

Buddha

You may be asking, "What's all this about my inner self? Is this a diet book or isn't it?" Confess it, the thought has crossed your mind, hasn't it?

You won't find no-cal, low-cal, low-sodium, low-carbohydrate, protein-sparing diets in these pages. You don't need them. You know what you have to eat to reach your natural weight. You've almost always known. Looking for just the right diet has become a game of postponing, a wish for magic. There are many reasonable, nutritious, health-producing, weight-reducing diets around. Which diet to follow is not your problem.

You have to learn to love your self enough to save your self. That's the answer, and always has been.

The answer lies within your reach; the medicine, the cure is in you. But when you cannot meet everyday problems, you lose confidence and look around for an escape. An overeater's unhappy escape is lurking behind the cold refrigerator door.

Your everyday frustrations will usually heal themselves if you do not overeat. It is that simple. You escape from the fat trap as you seek solutions from within rather than from outside yourself. You know that, don't you?

What have you done right today? You have questioned. Your mind is healthy and searching for answers. Where does the answer lie? Self-understanding. Say it again.

Today's Action Plan: I will choose one good diet plan and make it my "magic plan." I will light the lamp of self-understanding.

The Other Answer

*When faced with a problem . . . chances are the
solution lies not in a new idea but in a new look at an
old one.*

George Sheehan

There is a companion solution to chronic overweight,
because the same positive mental attitudes apply whether
you want to eat right or exercise.

There, it's out. The awful eight-letter word you can no
longer ignore. Only in recent years have we overweights
heard the experts say what we always knew but did not
understand: diets stop working after a certain point.
That's hardly a bombshell of information. We serious
dieters know that, don't we?

So the physical companion to the diet solution is
exercise to achieve the body you want. Why? Because
limiting food intake without adding exercise lowers the
body's "set point," and eventually makes dieting counter-
productive. In other words, the old yo-yo syndrome —
losing weight, only to bounce back to a higher weight —
is caused not just by overeating, but also by a low-
energy life.

The only way you can control your weight permanently is to eat a healthful diet and make exercise a daily
routine. And the road to this high-energy living, the
LifeWay of a winner, is paved with the bricks of self-
understanding. You see how it all comes together, don't
you?

What have you done right today? You have learned
that your body's chemistry adapts to low-calorie intake.
You know that exercise is the only way to raise your fat
set point, and stop the weight yo-yo. Get going.

**Today's Action Plan: I will do what has to be done
now. I will exercise.**

The High-energy Life

Nothing is too good to be true.
Ernest Holmes

Self-understanding, right diet, and exercise lead directly to the high-energy life. Won't it be wonderful to awake each morning to the reality of a thinner you? Won't it be great to face the day with enough energy to get the job done, make the team, win the day? Won't it?

To make a good habit, we must look to ourselves while our feet move toward what we want. No one deprives us of a thinner body but ourselves. Make it a habit to try new things, to work for your wants. What do you want? Wouldn't it be wonderful to have it?

Do you say, "I am ashamed of myself — I don't deserve anything better — I don't believe there is anything better for me in this world?" Nonsense!

Nothing is too good to be true. The best life you have ever thought about is not as good as the truth. Your imagination can conceive of only a fragment of what good can come to you. The thought that you can never have the high-energy life you want is just an old lie. Bury it. Reach for the best life you can conceive. Do it, won't you?

What have you done right today? You have caught a glimpse of what your life can be. After you put down the lie that you don't deserve better, you have seen that your wants can never exceed your possibilities.

Today's Action Plan: I will get rid of the old lies. I will believe that every good I can imagine can be true.

Why Self-esteem Is So Important

. . .self-schooled, self-scanned, self-honored, self-secure. . .
Matthew Arnold

Doing what we know needs to be done is the greatest builder of self-esteem. All the therapy, books, classes, parental love are nothing if we don't take action. People who have achieved their desires are achieving what they think they deserve; people who achieve nothing are doing the same thing. Be honest with yourself. Isn't that right?

Many people love you. They would give you the self-esteem you need, if they could. They may offer encouragement, rewards, even bribes. But they are helpless. The will to achieve doesn't come from the outside; it isn't handed to you or forced on you. The drive to win must come from within you.

Most of the world's people are non-achievers. They think success is luck, or a gift. A few people have the will, the drive to achieve. Aren't you happy to be part of this achieving minority?

What have you done right today? You found that you possess the will and drive to win. (You must or you wouldn't be reading this book.) You discovered that self-esteem is what powers your desire to win; and you know that your self-esteem builds as you do what you must do. This is the magic you've been waiting for.

Today's Action Plan: I will take charge of building my own self-esteem. From this minute on, I will be one of the minority of winners.

Perpetual Motion Engine

. . . still achieving, still pursuing . . .
Henry Wadsworth Longfellow

Achievement is the greatest motivator to achieve. Like a wonderful perpetual motion device, achievement continuously powers you to dare more, go higher, gain further success. You can fly! You'd rather fly high, wouldn't you?

Ah, but so many of us have excuses for not achieving. We call ourselves late bloomers, slow learners, and most of all, we have this awful handicap of overweight. Or wait, how about this one: "I don't have the time to do all this thinking and planning." Is that what you've said?

Time passes at the same rate for all of us; achievers use the same minutes, hours, and days that you use. Nothing is what you get for nothing. If you want a healthful, thinner body, a release from a horrible dependency on food, you must make the investment that is required. You are building for your future. Once you invest in yourself, it's not all uphill anymore; just getting into Action smooths the road ahead. You will get moving, won't you?

What have you done right today? You have decided that achievement is worth investing in today. You see that you can fly if you give up cherished excuses from the past. The past is gone. Today, you are an achiever.

Today's Action Plan: I will fly as high as I want to. I will achieve one thing that I have been postponing.

Self-esteem at Work

Oftentimes nothing profits more than self-esteem,
grounded on what is just and right.

John Milton

There are a few cruel people in the world, and there are others who are unthinking and insensitive. How many times has someone made a remark about your size? Maybe you were shopping for groceries and picked up an item, and a voice behind you said, "You shouldn't eat that!" What should you do?

If you thought of yourself only as a "weight," if you considered yourself an unworthy person, you may have believed you deserved this unpardonable intrusion. You might have explained, "This isn't for me, we're having company tonight." Why did you think you owed such a crude person an explanation? And yet how many times did you take insults, or answer intimate questions about your health, because you thought your weight had stripped you of the right to common courtesy?

You may have ignored the person and gone home feeling angry and depressed. But if you had a healthy sense of self-respect and a sense of inviolable worth, you could have turned and said: "That was a rude remark, and what I purchase is none of your business." If you can't manage a direct retort, try a five-second, icy stare.

Today you have a new, self-respecting LifeWay. Today you respond firmly to unmannerly remarks or gratuitous advice, or refuse to dignify them with notice. Good for you!

What have you done right today? You decided to never again accept discourteous attacks. Your weight is no one else's business.

Today's Action Plan: I will be self-respectful. I will insist that others — even imperfect strangers — treat me with respect.

Three Parts to a Whole

*You have to go as far as you can see . . . to see how far
you can go.*

Author unknown

You have resolved to turn your life around 180 degrees
so that you face a future unburdened by overeating
problems. At this point many overeaters turn to a diet, a
diet group, and a doctor. An excellent support trio. But
your new LifeWay must contain an additional and even
more powerful threesome: a weight-losing (later, a
weight-maintaining) food program, a physical fitness
program, and a mental fitness program. And it is
essential that you adopt all three parts of your new
program at once. You are developing your personal
three-part program, aren't you?

You were ill with a negative disease of the mind and
body. Sustained overeating and the resultant bouts of
grief, frustration, and panic impaired your physical and
mental systems. But now you have a positive new three-
part
cure. It's a triple injection of right-eating, physical
exercise, and mental fitness that attacks alien fat cells just
like antibodies seek out and destroy a life-threatening
virus.

Healthful eating, an energized body, and positive,
creative attitudes together produce healing through real
physical and biochemical changes. Believe in your ability
to make yourself well, won't you?

What have you done right today? You are engrossed
in a three-part positive plan for weight loss, physical
fitness, and mental fitness. You have everything you
need.

**Today's Action Plan: I will write all three parts of my
new plan on paper. I will commit myself to wellness.**

Watch Out for Self-criticism

By despising himself too much a man comes to be
worthy of his own contempt.
Henri Frederic Amiel

For the past two decades it has become a popular
pastime for people to participate in orgies of self-
criticism. By so doing, they try to rid their thinking of all
the mind-garbage they've collected. Perhaps you have
berated yourself publicly to show how psychologically
sensitive and knowledgeable you are. This is a wrong-
headed way of gaining approval. Stop it! No matter how
sincere, it has a negative impact on your self-image.
Right?

If our thoughts help us visualize ourselves, then how
much more do our spoken words influence others'
opinion of us, and our own? Have you ever spoken
about yourself to a companion, saying, for instance, "I'm
always so afraid in groups." Sometime later, your friend
parrots back to you, "Oh, you can't do that, you're
afraid in groups." Whammy! Double whammy! Your
spoken negative image (and, at that, it might not be
really true) judged you in another's mind and you had it
reinforced twice, by your own words and by your
friend's. You've made this mistake, haven't you?

What have you done right today? You have learned
about a destructive habit. You have seen that you must
speak positively. Remember, your own words are powerful weapons; use them to help yourself.

**Today's Action Plan: I will not play the self-criticism
game. I will reinforce the positive and powerful in me,
out loud.**

One Way Out

Admitting a problem is halfway to solution.
Anonymous

Are you having trouble admitting that you have a
weight problem? Are you still talking about baby fat, a
big frame, and glands? Until you admit you have a food
problem, that you are an overeater, you can't begin to
whip your weight problem. *The way to get out of
trouble is to first realize you're in trouble.* Unless you
perceive that you need help, you won't go to the lengths
necessary to help yourself. That makes sense, doesn't it?

If you don't see your pounds as your problem to
solve, you probably see yourself as a victim of fate;
somehow extra pounds just happen to you because the
world's picking on you again.

Victims have no fun and gain nothing but pounds and
pity. Who needs that? When overeaters can't admit their
problem and take charge of the solution, no one stops
the clock for them. The world leaves them behind.
Please don't let that happen to you. Say you won't.
Admit that you have a problem with food, then start
working on a solution. And do it now, won't you?

What have you done right today? You have learned
that you, and you alone, can make life work for you.
You are ready to admit that you have a problem. Good
for you!

Today's Action Plan: I admit that I have an eating
problem. I will follow a program of self-understanding,
eating, and exercise that will make my life work beautifully.

Feelings

Feelings are not reasons.

Alfred Adler

Do you use your feelings as an excuse not to do what you know you should do? Some people can't distinguish between what happens and how they feel about it. When you are disappointed, hurt, or angry, can you keep your perspective? Or do you say, "I feel so bad, I can't help eating." To be ruled by such feelings makes you a helpless victim of emotion. Like an electric wire on the loose, you snap from crisis to crisis, getting more scorched as you go. After a while, you lose the ability to tell genuine crisis from your emotional over-reaction. You can see how that could happen, can't you?

It's the old pain of self-pity again. Remembered hurts never die, never rest, they lurk there, ready to rationalize negative behavior. When you allow your feelings to be your reasons, you are like a baby, with no control, except to flail and cry and feel weak. There is nothing more frightening than to be helpless, to lose self-reliance, to never know what your feelings will drive you to next.

Feelings, used as reasons, are an alibi for not taking charge of your life. Thus, you'll function best if you keep a certain emotional distance between what happens to you and your reaction to it. Now you see it, don't you?

What have you done right today? You have learned the positive difference between reasons and feelings.

Today's Action Plan: No matter how bad I feel, I will not return to overeating. I will not allow self-pity to rule my emotions.

New Habits for Old

Forming a new habit is like winding string on a ball.
William James

It's nearly impossible to give up what you want to keep, so make sure you want to lose those extra pounds. Losing weight means forming a new habit of right-eating, a continuing process. It won't happen overnight. Give it time. The longer you wind the string William James talked about, the further ahead you'll be. If you drop it and it rolls, pick it up, and begin to wind again until the string is firmly attached to it. The stronger a new habit gets, the less compelling the temptation is to drop the ball. Don't you agree?

When you form the new habit of right-eating for health and attain that thinner, winner's body you want, the rewards are fantastic. Once you would have said, "I deserve to be fat," but no more. You see your worth because you are beginning to understand more about yourself.

What is your next weight goal? Write it down. If it's not written down where you can face it, it's not a goal. Writing is Action and every day you are putting Action into your life. You are a doer. You deserve applause, don't you? (Give yourself a hand!)

What have you done right today? You have learned that new habits just don't happen, you make them happen. You have decided to "wind string" until your new habit of right-eating becomes stronger than the old habit of overeating.

Today's Action Plan: I will make good new habits stronger every day. I will follow the Twelve Action MindSteps as a doer, not a regretter.

For Me — Right Now!

*If I am not for me, then who is for me; and if not now,
then when?*

Hillel

It's too late now for you to go back to your self-
destructive ways. You know too much, you've come too
far. By now, you have learned a new way of thinking,
and most important of all, gained self-understanding
which compels you to go forward. You are for you,
because who else can take charge of your life, right now?
If not now, then when?

Yesterday is a cancelled check; tomorrow is but a
promissory note. The past is buried; today you are
beginning your future. This minute should be one of the
happiest of your life because you are getting rid of a
curse, the compulsion to overeat, using food destructive-
ly.

The more you understand, the harder it will be for
you to turn around and go back to the negative rational-
izations you once made; all the tired excuses you had
just won't work anymore. Self-knowledge has detoured
any overeating pleasure you once might have had.

Sorry. You're stuck with self-reliance, with health,
with achievement and happiness. Nothing can stop you
from achieving, if that is what you want. You're relieved
about that, aren't you?

What have you done right today? You have learned
that the road ahead to achievement is really easier than
the road back to overeating.

**Today's Action Plan: I will walk on. I will enjoy this
day because I am for me, and right now.**

Don't Use this Book as an Excuse

*If you don't want to do something, one excuse is as good
as another.*

Yiddish Saying

Some overweights have found outside help to lose and
keep off excess weight. Their help may come from a
weight-losing group, a doctor, a spa, or a spiritual
advisor. If you have such a support system and it's
working, fine! If so, you may think it unnecessary to use
the Twelve Action MindSteps and read this book.
Perhaps, but consider this: the be-all of every weight-loss
or maintenance program is motivation, and it's difficult
for any overeater to get enough motivation on a day-to-
day basis. Either the group isn't meeting, the doctor is
playing golf, or the spa is closed. Even our spiritual
advisor takes a vacation at times. That's what both *Thin
Books* give you, a friend at hand, some straight talk,
someone who knows how you feel, every time you need
a boost. You can see how it can help, can't you?

You may even think that this book's emphasis on self-
understanding is selfish. But please be honest with yourself. If you can't take charge of your own life, how much
can you give to others?

As for the other help techniques you've allowed into
your weight-loss program: who do you think made the
decision to let them in and let them stay? That's one of
the greatest take-charge decisions of all, isn't it?

What have you done right today? There are many
ways you can help yourself, and you're doing one of
them right now: you are reading this book and getting
into Action. Keep it up every day.

**Today's Action Plan: I will take all the help I can get.
I will add the Twelve Action MindSteps to whatever
other help I have in my life.**

Who We Are

Character is a victory, not a gift.

Anonymous

Action is character; we are what we do. We can talk about what we will do someday, but unless what we say agrees with what we do, it is meaningless. Talking endlessly about what we want, without ever moving our feet in harmony with our mouths, is just wasting time. Soon people don't believe us, and we don't believe ourselves. Sad, isn't it?

In a way, idle talk and addiction are much the same. They are both means of avoiding action. Did you ever think of an addiction to overeating, or to certain foods, as a way of evading life's demands? Addiction to food and talking-instead-of-doing are two sides of the same coin.

You say, "That's unfair. I really do have big plans; I'm just waiting for the right time to come along." Of course you try to believe it, to cushion the pain of living a low-energy, non-achieving life. But have you fooled yourself with this alibi?

What you do is what you truly mean. There is only one way to live — in direct, toe-to-toe contact with today. It's tough, but you can do it, can't you?

What have you done right today? You learned that to be a winner, you must act. You are aware that you, and you alone, can change your life. Don't have it any other way.

Today's Action Plan: I will not be caught in the trap of talking instead of doing. I will follow the eighth Action MindStep and do whatever has to be done.

Are You Rolling a Rock Uphill?

Every time you act, you add strength to the motivating idea behind what you've done.

George Weinberg

In Greek mythology, Sisyphus was a king condemned by Zeus to roll a stone to the top of a hill. All day, he rolled it toward the top, but when he stopped at night, the stone rolled to the bottom of the hill again. Sisyphus was doomed to roll his stone up the hill every day. Does that sound like the story of your life?

Overeating is like the burden of the Sisyphus stone.

A new life, one that fires you away from your no-win dependence, won't come easily; it would be the greatest self-deception to believe that you can change habits of mind and appetite without effort. That doesn't mean life is an endless fight for survival. There's loveliness and beauty in living free of your compulsion.

Soon positive new habits will overwhelm your negative old habits. Once the new habits of eating and thinking take over, your Sisyphus stone will stay at the top of your mountain, and so will you. That's a promise. Persistence is the key. You know that, don't you?

What have you done right today? You have committed yourself to a healthful, winner's life. Whatever it takes, you know you will provide yourself with the desire to succeed. It's the best decision you've ever made.

Today's Action Plan: I will win and be thin. By eating right one day at a time, I will stay on top of the mountain forever.

MindSteps

It is impossible to underrate human intelligence.
Henry Adams

The ideas embodied in the Twelve Action MindSteps are
for you. They were designed to lift you up, to open your
mind to all the possibilities that you have buried for so
long behind a barrier of flesh. They present the positive,
take-charge life. Each MindStep is a principle that lifts
you to a higher level of self-understanding. Study them.
Know them. Own them. You can do that, can't you?

You say, "I tried something like this a few months
ago, but it didn't work. I'm still as fat and unhappy as
ever." Is that what you're saying?

Today, you are another person. Science tells us that
there is not one atom of your body that was a part of us
even a few months ago. Changes occur every day. Some
part of you is born anew today, and will be born anew
tomorrow. Your yesterdays have no power over you
unless you allow them the power.

What was true a few months ago, was true for a
different person. Today you are developing the unique
human being that you are. Your confidence is growing.
You have a desire and want to get into Action. Do you
see now what a very different person you've become?

What have you done right today? You have refused to
allow yesterday's failure to punish the winning new
person you have become. You are willing to give
yourself a fresh new start everyday.

**Today's Action Plan: I will use the MindSteps as a
stairway to a higher understanding of myself. I will give
this new me every possible chance.**

The Greatest Forgiveness

To err is human, to forgive, divine.
Alexander Pope

In this often-quoted line, you probably think Pope was talking about forgiving other people, and perhaps he was. But there is another forgiveness, a greater, even more divine forgiveness that you haven't practiced: self-forgiveness. No weight can be heavier than your inability to forgive yourself for getting fat, and nothing is more tragic than living day after day with self-hatred in your heart. That's so, isn't it?

Self-hate causes you to berate yourself to others. You say, "I'll never be able to stick to this diet," and then you make your prediction come true. The cycle spirals endlessly: self-hate, self-berate, overate.

There is only one way to fight your way out of your own trap: *forgive yourself!* There is no way you can live a high-energy, Action-oriented, achieving life, until you practice self-forgiveness. It's one of the most creative acts overeaters can accomplish, and the foundation for a life that knows more joy than pain, more success than failure. And you must forgive yourself again and again. A hundred thousand times if necessary. Say YES to that, won't you?

What have you done right today? You see that you need to forgive yourself, to deny that failure-image, and accept the intelligent, lovable, winning you. You have learned that you first must give yourself a chance, before you could possibly give anything to another person. Now, that's divine!

Today's Action Plan: I will find a new love. It will be me.

February 23

Have the Time of Your Life

*Time is no speedway between the cradle and the grave
but space to find a place in the sun.*
Phil Bosmans

It's never going to be today again; that's the essence of
the eighth Action MindStep. That means you should live
in this moment and don't waste a moment. It does not
mean you shouldn't plan for the future, just don't worry
about it. Planning is Action, whereas worrying is a
passive victim's game. Work against procrastination.
Postponing living is like stealing from yourself. Who
wants a life devoted to killing time? You want more
from life, don't you?

Yes, you want to live every moment as fully, as
serenely, as possible. Only then will you have the
courage to change and the wisdom to believe that you
can. But don't move so fast that you have no time to
enjoy your own success. And with one weight goal at a
time, you are going to have a lot of success.

Time is a gift, a precious gift, to use as you want.
How to spend it is your choice. Aren't you astonished
that you have the ability and time to achieve your own
place in the sun?

Learn to love knowledge and change, and time will
not drag, but will race along. Give yourself some time to
laugh and to dance. You have earned it. Give yourself
some of that kind of time today, won't you?

What have you done right today? Your time is so full
of positive things that you know you are alive. You see
that you can do astonishing, unique things with the
minutes and hours of your day. Have the time of your
life!

**Today's Action Plan: I will not kill time. I will take
the gift of time and use it.**

The Pain in Gain Is Mainly in the Brain

*People will say the pain was all in my mind, which is
true. But that's the worst place to have it.*
Maury Wills

Face it. When you get up enough courage to get on the
scales after a weight gain, you're not hurting anywhere
but in your self-esteem. Those hated new pounds mean
you've cheated yourself. You ask the great "why" question: "Why don't I do what I know I must do?"

The reason you don't is that your push is in conflict
with your shove; you push forward your desire to be
thin and your anxieties shove back — hard. Result:
weight gain. Sadly, this is true, isn't it?

Go ahead and face pain!

What? You've always avoided pain, maybe with an
extra snack or two. Don't do it, not only because you'll
gain weight, but because that pain can teach. You leap
away from your pain far too easily, so nothing comes of
it; you don't learn from it. That's too bad, because pain's
lesson is that you don't like pain. Once this lesson is
learned, pain becomes your resource and your ally. Ask
yourself: "How much pain do I need before I've had
enough? Now, am I ready to look at life beyond excess
food?" If your answer is YES, say "yes," out loud. You're
beginning to suspend your disbelief, aren't you?

What have you done right today? You have learned
that your suffering and conflict are an essential part of
being. Once you are willing to experience and take the
responsibility for the pain of overeating, you are ready
to push forward to the body you most desire.

Today's Action Plan: I will accept my pain and
understand its lesson. I will practice pushing my desire
for a healthy new body past my anxieties.

Today Is "Some Day"

[When you were young] you were always full of the future: some day you are going to do this. And some day is here or it's never going to be here. It's frightening, as if a needle got stuck in the record of life.
Cynthia Ozick

Pay attention to today. No matter what your age is now — young, or old, or in-between — today is vital. In this hectic, busy world, there are so many demands on your time that you must set priorities. Overeaters like to put themselves at the bottom of their priority list. Do you do this?

Always make time for the things you want for you. If you don't, depression and overeating can wreck even the busiest day. How many times have you promised yourself, "When I have more time, I'll start a good diet and exercise program."

You will never have more time than you do today. No one else has any more hours and minutes than you do, yet some people find time to lead the high-energy life you'd like for yourself. Paradoxically, the more they attend to their wants, the more they can accomplish for themselves and for others. They don't *make* more time, they simply use what they have. You may think you are too busy to pay attention to your eating problem, but you spend more time agonizing, rationalizing, and self-pitying, than you admit. Truthfully, isn't that so?

What have you done right today? You have looked at the often painful ways you lose precious time, time you can't afford to waste. You have decided that today is that once far-off "some day."

Today's Action Plan: I will use all the time I have for accomplishment. I will not wait for "some day." I'll pay attention to me now.

Why?

The cause of obesity could be almost anything.
Dr. Albert Stunkard

Every overweight person has dealt with the question, "Why me?" There isn't an overweight alive who doesn't know someone who eats twice as much and weighs half as much. That's true, isn't it?

Overweight is complex. Some people have too many fat cells or fat cells that are too large, or both. Some people become overweight as children, others as adults. Some people eat too much, others eat the right amount but have bodies that use calories too slowly. Overweights come in every size, with mild, moderate, and severe weight problems.

What's the cause? It could be hormones, genes, personality, or the modern world of convenience that makes food readily available to inactive people. It could be any of these reasons, all of them, an unknown factor, or a combination of X-factors. It isn't fair. But don't expect fair. That's a failure's waiting game. You're not going to wait, are you?

Just because you may be predisposed to overweight, doesn't mean you have to *be* overweight. It will be wonderful when science finds the fat-producing "bug," virus, gene or hormone, and develops the magic cure — a pill, shot, or operation. Until then, try these remedies: right-eating for your individual body, exercise to improve your fat-converting capacity, and positive MindSteps. You need to live a richer life now, not to wait for an uncertain "cure," don't you?

What have you done right today? You've faced your overweight problem, no matter how unfair it is, and taken charge.

Today's Action Plan: I will live fully right now, building a new LifeWay that works. I won't worry about what's fair; instead, I'll concentrate on what's necessary.

How Winners Take Rejection

What lies behind us and what lies before us are tiny matters compared with what lies within us.
William Morrow

How do you take rejection? Do you feel as if you have been personally attacked? Do you slink away to nurse your wounds, and then go on a food binge to get even with the rejector? After your binge, does your anger turn to self-loathing? You've played this self-destructive game, haven't you?

That's why the first Action MindStep is so important. Unless you develop a solid understanding of your unique worth, you are prey for every rejector who comes along. Why allow yourself to be knocked this way and that? If you know your unique worth, you can handle rejection or criticism without hiding behind excess food.

Winners don't take rejection personally. They fight rejection by trying again and again, for as long as it takes. They solve the problem if they can; then they forget it and walk on. What's done is done. With this attitude, *you may be rejected, but you cannot be defeated.*

No one else is in charge of your happiness. Don't let others destroy your happiness and, for goodness sake, don't cooperate with them if they try. Most people aren't out to ruin you. They're merely rejecting an idea, an invitation, or an offer, not you. You do understand that, don't you?

What have you done right today? You have learned the way winners handle rejection. Winners find a positive side

to rejection; they see it as an opportunity to change others' ideas about themselves. Go ahead, show them!

Today's Action Plan: I will not take rejection personally. I will accept my unique worth so that rejection will simply seem like another challenge, another way to win.

Questions

"The question is," said Humpty Dumpty, "which is to be master — that's all."

Lewis Carroll

Have you been reading *The Thin Book II* out loud? There's a very good reason for doing so. You've probably noticed that as each day's reading progresses, you are asked questions that often end with the words, "isn't it?" "don't you?" or "won't you?" Sales professionals call these phrases *tie-downs,* and they ask them to elicit YES answers from prospects. Look back over the tie-downs on previous pages and see if you answered YES to most of them. You did, didn't you?

The sales technique is to get the prospect to answer a series of minor YESes so that when it's time to sell the product, the prospect has been conditioned all along to answer YES. Without being aware of it, you've been both salesperson and sales prospect all these weeks.

At this point, you may say, "I get it. You've been trying to sell me on myself." You're absolutely right! Nice to be right, isn't it?

"Wait a minute," you may say. "Why tell me the trick? Now that I know about it, it won't work any longer." Wrong. It will work twice as well. Every time you read a tie-down, you will know you should react positively. Like a computer, you are programmed. From now on when you get to this part of each day's reading, you will be ready to buy the product, a thinner and happier life. You're ready, aren't you?

What have you done right today? You have learned that there is a YES system at work in these pages, and that its

purpose is to sell you on what a wonderfully unique individual you are.

Today's Action Plan: I will say YES to a positive life. I will buy my own product.

March 1

Amazing Grace

I have been all my life in hiding.
                                                    Kate Millett

In the hymn "Amazing Grace," one joyous line could be a theme song for the recovering overeater. "I once was lost, but now am found." When you take charge of your eating and your life, it's like being found — but even more, it's like coming out of hiding. You know that feeling, don't you?

You have been lonely. When we hide from ourselves, we don't want to know ourselves. There is no greater loneliness. In trying to find comfort, you became dependent on food, and found only misery. You became lost.

But things are different now. Every day you are finding your way back to life. You have come out of hiding. You know that anyone who wants to climb out of the pit of loneliness can do so, using the Action MindSteps to self-understanding. It is hard to believe that it could be that simple. But to gain belief, you need only give up your unbelief.

When you come out of hiding and take charge of your life, your loneliness will disappear and along with it your addiction to overeating. Eating excessively was one way to ward off loneliness. Deep in your heart, you knew that, didn't you?

What have you done right today? You have decided never to hide from yourself again. Your eating and exercise plan for a winning life is your statement of belief. Hooray for you!

Today's Action Plan: I will give up my unbelief in my ability to win. I will never hide again.

Anger

The only way to make me feel better, was to make everyone else feel worse.
                    Overeaters Anonymous member

When you're overweight in a thin-is-in society, you can fall victim to helpless rage. Some of us live with a perpetual silent scream. "Somebody's going to pay for this," is our battle cry. Have you ever secretly felt like this?

Often compulsive overeaters harbor an unconscious wish for revenge, an indirectly expressed aggression born of anger and resentment against others, but mostly against themselves.

We appear to be vindictive with others — family, friends, co-workers — but if the truth were known, our behavior is just another way of getting even with ourselves for the awful way we feel about overeating. It's true, others suffer, but oh, how we stagger under the burden of self-hate. Far too often, "getting even" for overeaters means plunging headlong into despair. We become our own worst punishers.

No one needs to be punished, least of all you. That's the big point. Forget about getting even. Instead, get thinner, healthier, more successful. That's the way winners look at life. Anger takes too much energy away from what you really want to do. Doesn't how you feel about what you do determine how you feel about yourself? Say YES.

What have you done right today? You have replaced the
    silent scream of anger with constructive Action. You see that it is far more fun to reach out for the good life than to punish yourself for the past. About time, too.

Today's Action Plan: I will avoid angry conflict. I will feel only positive things about myself.

March 3

How to Avoid Success

Tall trees take a lot of wind.
Flemish Saying

Here's a sure-fire method to avoid success: never attempt anything. Never try any of the Twelve Action Mind-Steps; never try to take charge of your life. You can avoid success forever just by never trying. This is the way we protect ourselves from failure, isn't it?

Are you hiding from possible failures? Are you afraid to grow tall because you might not be able to "take the wind?" You don't always win. Maybe not the first time, nor even the second. Be prepared for that. You are trying to do the toughest thing in this world, lower your food intake and increase your energy expenditure until you achieve and maintain your desired weight. Hunger, like breathing, is a basic biological drive. What you like to eat is very personal. But you are developing a new attitude about overeating: you aren't "giving up" extra food, but "getting rid of" negative behavior. It's difficult, but, yes, you can win.

Winners could paraphrase Benjamin Franklin's advice on trying with: "If at first you don't succeed, fail, fail again." You see how challenging that feisty attitude is, don't you?

What have you done right today? You have decided not to avoid failure, because avoiding it means never trying. Though your hunger may be powerful, your desire for a new take-charge way of living is even more powerful. If you say so, it's true.

Today's Action Plan: I will stand tall and take a chance. I will keep trying until I succeed.

Changing

If you're never scared or embarrassed or hurt,
it means you never take any chances.

Julia Sorel

Change inevitably means that part of your comfortable old self must die to give birth to your new winning self. Sometimes we suffer from labor pains. We can't just relax and let the needed change take over; we fight to keep our familiar overeating ways. It's all part of a complex grief process. But we overeaters — when faced with the visual, emotional, and spiritual results of our overeating — know that we *must* change. Remember that success "loves" those who change. You want to be loved by success, don't you?

The eleventh Action MindStep teaches: **don't fight inevitable change;** make change work for you by facing life's problems honestly and working your way through the emotional thickets. Keep the best of yourself. Then get rid of your negative, destructive habits.

Does that sound tough? Are you saying, "I'm too weak-willed to change"? It's become fashionable in recent years to demean the idea of strength of will, but if strength of will didn't exist, nothing would be accomplished. Remember, too, that your own strength of will can be made up of many strengths, including your faith in a Higher Power and the support of friends and professional advisers. From whatever sources you have constructed your strength of will, you demonstrated it when you decided to take charge of your life, didn't you?.

What have you done right today? You have learned that you are strong-willed. You are determined to face your fear of change so you can make change work for you. And you can do it, too!

Today's Action Plan: I will begin to make whatever changes are necessary in my life. I have the strength and the will to do it.

March 5

Be Environment-conscious

*Food is the cheapest and most abundant mood-altering
drug on the market.*

Anne Scott Beller

Don't keep your binge food handy either in your house
or in your office. Don't loiter in bakeries or candy shops.
Make a simple rule: if you don't want to eat it, don't
have it available. Foods — especially our binge foods —
are all around us, on every television program, menu,
and magazine cover. It's impossible to get rid of these
temptations completely, but you can take steps to minimize their influence. You can see how helpful that would
be, can't you?

Be honest about the environment you create. Don't
kid yourself that you buy your binge food for your
children, your roommate, or your guests. When you
stock up on low-control foods, you're creating a negative
environment

If you don't want to slip, "avoid slippery places," as
the book *A Day at a Time* warns. Don't turn your own
kitchen into the food equivalent of an opium den. It's
like living with a clanging fire alarm; there's no peace.
Keep the junk food out of your environment, won't you?

What have you done right today? You have realized
that achievers structure a safe dieting environment by
avoiding binge foods. You know that your home must
be a safe place to live, grow, and change.

**Today's Action Plan: I will binge-proof my environ-
ment. I will stay away from slippery places.**

Memories

God gave us memories so that we might have roses in December.

James M. Barrie

Overweights store some of the worst memories: cruel rejections, body-embarrassments, lost jobs, chances never taken or never offered — you are filled with negative memories. It's true, they've happened, but they're gone. Let go of those memories of yourself as a pudgy child, fat adolescent, and overweight adult. Don't nurse these destructive thoughts — kick them out! You'd enjoy that, wouldn't you?

Your memory holds the accumulated knowledge of your past, everything that ever happened to you. If the memory is pleasant, cherish it; if it's painful, throw it out. What you can do today is take charge of your *future* memories.

Every day you make memories. Funnel today's experiences into tomorrow's happy reflections. If you are committed to a winning life, you have also put yourself in charge of your memories so that they will be a resource in your tomorrows. Make confident, committed, sunny, winning memories. Do that, won't you?

What have you done right today? You have taken charge of how memory works for you. You have discovered how your commitment puts you in control of your future memories. Start building them now.

Today's Action Plan: I will let go of negative memories. For the future, I will begin to make positive memories.

People Who Need People

"My people," my soul cried. "Who are my people?"
Rosa Zagnoni Marinoni

Some overeaters need to share their recovery process
with other overeaters. Fine! There are several international groups: Overeaters Anonymous, Weight Watchers, Take Off Pounds Sensibly (TOPS), and numerous
local groups. If you are a person who needs other
people, decide which group is best for you, and join. Do
it today, won't you?

There's a practical reason for you to consider joining a
group: they work. Groups tend to have higher recovery
rates than lone dieters. Why? Because they have a
supportive, accepting environment. They give you a
specific way to view your weight problem, which ends
confusion and helps you focus your energy. They help
you learn about yourself so you can understand your
problem better. They show you it is possible to win and
you can identify with the winners.

Take all the help you can get. That's the idea. Chances
are that, like many overeaters, you are a loner. Overeating led you to isolate yourself from others. After the
initial contact with the group you'll find yourself looking
forward to meetings — to stimulation, knowledge and
camaraderie. It's a strange paradox: you can get more
help from a stranger who overeats than from those who
know you best but can't understand the reason you use
food as you do. Such understanding is worth searching
for, isn't it?

What have you done right today? You see many good
reasons for giving a group of fellow overeaters a chance.
The "buddy system" provides the support you need.

**Today's Action Plan: I will attend a group meeting. I
will seek and accept help for my overeating problem.**

Gifts

*Those gifts are ever the most acceptable which the giver
has made precious.*

Ovid

Are you good to yourself, not indulgent, but loving, as
to a friend? Do you give yourself little gifts to show your
love: a gentle word, a walk in the leaves? Do you find a
closer contact with your Higher Power? Do you criticize
yourself little, encourage much, and forgive quickly? If
that's not the way you treat yourself, you'd like to,
wouldn't you?

To be a whole person, you can't separate your
spiritual self and your physical body, for it's within your
body that your unique spirit lives. All of this is deeply
significant for the winner you are. It is a part of your
daily contemplation, isn't it?

Also, give a gift of yourself to someone else, some
other overeater who needs your special understanding.
Schedule some of your time, money, and effort into
your family, neighborhood or community — something
beyond your self and your desires. Yours is a battered
spirit. To build a winner's strength, you need to build
your sense of personal worth. Nothing clears away the
debris of past failure like doing something to make
others glad that you were there.

At any given moment, do the most productive, positive thing you can do, including moments of caring for
your spiritual self. You do understand that, don't you?

What have you done right today? You have seen that
you cannot neglect your spiritual self. You know that
you can endure anything, so long as your unconquerable
spirit is nourished.

**Today's Action Plan: I will nurture my spirit. I will
nurture others through service until my spirit glows.**

Are You a "Never Enougher"?

It is curious what shifts we make to escape thinking.
Herman Melville

Some overeaters never get enough — not just of food, but of life. Nothing — no matter what quantity or quality — is ever enough. They always have a feeling of deprivation. Isn't that sad?

People who feel deprived, no matter how fortunate they really are, need to become self-nurturers. They need more self-acceptance and less self-criticism.

Above all, they need to stop disqualifying emotional support and comfort from others. Too often, never-enoughers not only don't care about themselves, but they won't allow others to get close enough to care.

It will be difficult at first, but deliberately choose friends who are affectionate by nature. You know the kind: they sympathize, they're touchers, they'll even cuddle you if they're encouraged. These are important people to you because they meet your need to feel connected to others emotionally. They not only help you to feel loved, but lovable.

The world is rich with love, and you deserve your share. Just reach out, won't you?

What have you done right today? You discarded the feeling that there is never enough for you. You accepted nurturing from yourself and others to replace false feelings of deprivation.

Today's Action Plan: I will not be a "never-enougher." I will reach out for the emotional support I need.

Why Not Today?

I can promise you that you'll begin to enjoy your workout.

Dr. Kenneth H. Cooper

It's not easy. Overweight people who begin an exercise program face problems that never concern our thinner brothers and sisters. For example, clothing manufacturers never dream that a woman beyond size 14 would pick up a tennis racket, so suitable clothing is unavailable. Just the thought of appearing in leotards has probably stopped more overweights from exercising than any other reason. Bluntly put, exercise can be a source of embarrassment for the overweight, can't it?

But embarrassment isn't an excuse for not working toward a high-energy body. Be ingenious. Don't squeeze into a too-tight jogging suit, hear someone laugh at you, and suddenly give up fitness — all in one morning. You've got two better choices: ignore the insensitive clod and head for the gym, or start your exercise program at home. Then when you begin to firm and tune-up your body, you'll have enough exercise success to overrun any vestiges of embarrassment. A little success is a great motivator.

Start exercising. There are dozens of good books and cassettes on the subject. Get one. Do it today. Use that exercycle gathering dust in the garage. Have a little exercise success today and you'll have more tomorrow. But you have to make a start, don't you? Say YES. Say YES again.

What have you done right today? You have decided that nothing will keep you from the high-energy, winning life that you deserve.

Today's Action Plan: I will not let anything stop me from achieving fitness. Today, I will exercise my body so that I can be in the running.

March 11

Wrong Path

Don't look back; something could be gainin' on you.
Satchel Paige

Looking back might mean you haven't defined your next goal. Unclear goals can make you feel wary, as if you're being followed by an unidentified pursuer. Know who that is? It's you. The old negative you, scared and calling out, "You're taking a chance going forward. Wait for me!" Have you ever heard that voice from the past?

Clearly define your goals all along the way. In MindStep nine you decided to set a series of weight-loss goals. Think of each goal as a hand reaching to pull you forward. Write your goals down. That helps. Make a plan to achieve them — whether it's joining a weight-losing group or fellowship, asking a doctor's help, or helping yourself — but make a real plan. Go after results.

Don't look back unless that's the path you want to take. Don't listen to nay-saying voices. You know where you want to go — forward. That's true, isn't it?

What have you done right today? You have learned that only through planning and persistence can you make dreams come true. You have reaffirmed the Action MindStep that tells you to aim for achievable weight goals. Easy does it, but do it. Now that's smart!

Today's Action Plan: I will look ahead on the path to achievement. I will make a plan and aim straight for it.

Work, Success, and Exercise

The high tension and low activity of modern life make a deadly mixture.

Dr. Kenneth H. Cooper

There is ample frustration living overweight in a thin-is-best world. But couple it with a high-tension job and you see how an overweight can be in emotional trouble. Then add to this deadly duo debilitating inactivity fostered by a culture which invented the electric egg-beater. You see that tension and inactivity are your powerful foes, don't you?

You know that exercise leads to a fit body and emotional well-being. However, did you know that exercise can help you advance on the job?

Recent research, compiled by the Illinois Council on Health and Physical Fitness, reveals that: absenteeism drops by 60 percent among people who are actively involved in an exercise program; exercisers score 70 percent higher in decision-making skills; and 60 percent more of them enjoy their work more than the non-exercisers do. That's not all. A survey by Canada Life Insurance Company shows that exercisers aren't job-hoppers; sedentary employees average ten times more turnover.

Some companies now are making substantial investments in equipment and incentives to get their employees off their "bottom lines." Don't you think you ought to put your energy where the smart money is going? Exercise today.

What have you done right today? You have been receptive to new information about exercise. You're going to exercise today, not just for your "bottom line" (success in your job), but for your life.

Today's Action Plan: I will reduce tension in my life with exercise. I will make an exercise investment.

Curiosity

Be one of those upon whom nothing is lost.
Henry James

Winners are curious about life, about the ordinary as well as the extraordinary, the inner as well as the outer world. The more winners know, the more options they have, and the fuller and richer their life can be. You'd like to be that kind of person, wouldn't you?

But knowledge is only the beginning. To accomplish great things you must also be ready to act on what you know. Knowledge is the foundation, and Action is the castle you can build upon it. Yes, you can. You know you can.

Learn good nutrition. Learn about aerobic exercise. Learn to have a sense of "wellness." Pursue knowledge that will carry you to your dream's fulfillment. Every day you gain more knowledge, you gain more power to attain your dream. You don't need magic to believe in yourself. Believing *is* the magic.

Remember, winning is supported by Action, and Action is activated by knowledge. Actually, Action is senseless without knowledge. You believe this, don't you? Say YES. There, you're getting smarter (and thinner) every day, aren't you?

What have you done right today? You see that new ideas encourage decisions, inform actions, and discourage self-deception. You know now that knowledge opens the world, so you can choose from so many more options.

Today's Action Plan: I will absorb knowledge like a sponge. I will put this knowledge into Action and win.

A Different Grief

Grief may be joy misunderstood.
                              Elizabeth Barrett Browning

Overweights may go through two different grief process-
es. When we're covered with excess flesh, we grieve for
the person and body we want to be. The longer we've
been overweight the more we feel this grief. Psychology
explains it as an alienation from the self, but it feels more
like grief to the overweight. It's like grieving for a
prisoner, falsely imprisoned. You understand this grief,
don't you?

After weight loss there's another kind of grief mingled
with confused feelings of fear and sadness at the loss of a
part of one's self. We lose our sense of identity and get
confused. The newly thin person reaches back for that
familiar self and sometimes gains weight again.

There is a way to sidestep this destructive weight-loss
grief experience, or at least to minimize it. Redefine
yourself as your weight goes down; don't wait. Working
the MindSteps in this book is part of the redefinition
process. Are you learning to think and act like a thinner
winner — now — so you'll be ready for the essential you
that begins to emerge? Say YES to that. Out loud. Listen
to your own voice affirm yourself, won't you?

What have you done right today? You know that if
you "get rid of" your extra weight instead of "losing" it,
you will head off any misplaced grief when your new
body appears.

**Today's Action Plan: I will get rid of my weight. I will
understand that any grief I feel is misunderstood joy.**

Personal Best

When the horse is dead, get off.
Kirk M. Sorensen

You're losing weight regularly and you feel great. You are honestly following your eating plan, exercising, building your winning attitude. You're doing everything you've done right along, but suddenly your efforts don't show in pounds lost. You've hit a plateau. What now? Too often in the past, the answer has been to recede into self-pity and say, "Look at that scale! I'm doing everything I should but I'm not getting thinner. To heck with it, I might as well eat!" Have you ever felt that way?

If you're stuck, change something. Act! It doesn't matter what you change — adjust your diet, or add a new exercise — the important thing is to take charge. Act on your determination and desire to reach your goal.

Winning athletes always try to top their best. You'll never know what your capacities are until you try. Nothing comes from nothing; something comes from something. Go out on a limb. The greatest idea you can get from these pages is: there is no failure but quitting. Winners never quit, and you're a winner, aren't you?

What have you done right today? You have learned you can win despite setbacks, if you act on what you know. Also, a want is just a wish until you make it happen by planning, persistence, and your determination to win.

Today's Action Plan: If I am stuck, I will change something. I will always be capable of bettering my past record.

Fear

*Fear of becoming a has-been keeps some people from
becoming anything.*

Eric Hoffer

Are you a worry machine? If so, probably half your
fears begin with the words, "what if." With these words
you turn opportunity into difficulty. Some concerns are
legitimate, but don't inflate them. In the past you've
worried unnecessarily, haven't you?

When you're afraid that something might happen, you
must make plans to deal with that possibility. All right,
let's do an exercise. Think of the worst possibility. Now
outline all the steps to prevent it from happening, to fix
it if it does happen, or to live with it if you can't fix it.
Do that now.

Do you see what you've done? While you were
problem-solving, you shut off the worry machine.

Now that you've learned how to deal with your worry
machine, you can walk on to a more positive attitude.
Plan, anticipate, and work toward your future instead of
worrying about it. Wouldn't you prefer to live this way?

What have you done right today? You have learned
better ways of dealing with the future than worrying
about it. You've taken charge of your worst possible
"what if?" so it has no power to haunt you.

Today's Action Plan: I will turn off my worry
machine. No matter what I fear, I will deal with it
instead of eating over it.

One Way to Achieve

*If you want to change what other people think of you,
you must change what you think of yourself.*
George Bernard Shaw

Are you trying to get everyone to like you? If so, the problem isn't with others, but with you. You are basing your self-acceptance on others' opinions. It's fun to be popular, it's nice to be appreciated, but it's not absolutely necessary for self-esteem. Remember self-acceptance can't be given to you, but is built from within because you approve of your own Action. That makes sense, doesn't it?

Beware from whom you seek approval. If you seek it from someone who finds your success threatening, you're asking for trouble. Your weight loss might be extremely threatening to those closest to you. They may see you changing and fear you will force change on them. You won't be "good old fat so-and-so," someone of no consequence. Now they must deal with a powerful person, a winner with positive attitudes whom they may even secretly envy and unknowingly try to sabotage.

Self-acceptance is the state of being your own person, self-reliant, not dependent on others. Think of how wonderful that will be for you and others too. Think about it, won't you?

What have you done right today? You have stopped thinking that self-acceptance involves acceptance by others.

Today's Action Plan: I will accept myself as a thinner winner. I will not let anyone change me back.

Have Fun

Against the assault of laughter, nothing can stand.
                                        Mark Twain

Winners know how to have fun. True, they are achievers first, but rest and recreation are essential to the positive, productive rhythms of their lives. A valuable machine isn't allowed to run until it breaks down for lack of time off or maintenance, is it?

Treat yourself well. Program fun and relaxation into your day along with work, right-eating, and exercise. You must release pent-up frustration and pressure so that tension doesn't lead to overeating. Tension may have no single cause, but may be an accumulation of little irritations that can grow into a big problem without a non-food escape valve.

Take time now to schedule some fun. Fun may be reading, or working on a hobby, or being with friends. Call a friend. Socialize. Turn on your natural charm; adopt a bright and cheerful attitude. Make your fun pure pleasure, by not mixing it with business. Soon you'll find your stress (and more pounds) melting away. Remember, though, fun is low-calorie; it doesn't always mean going out to dinner, does it?

What have you done right today? You have learned that relaxation and fun are an essential part of the achiever's life. Put your feet up (or get them to a dance floor). Enjoy!

Today's Action Plan: Today I will include some fun for my well-being. After relaxing, I will be renewed.

Become Your Own Nutritionist

Jack Sprat could eat no fat
his wife could eat no lean
and so between the two of them
they licked the platter clean.

Mother Goose

The Sprats knew what they couldn't eat, and you have also learned what to avoid to reach and maintain your healthy weight. Now it's time for you to learn more about how certain nutritional elements work in your body, and why. You can learn by going to a professional nutritionist or doing your own nutritional research. You need to become your own positive nutritionist because you're the one on the front lines, aren't you?

You need to know about nutrients and how they work for you. You're responsible for that; nobody else is.

Once you know how food works in conjunction with organs and glands, you'll learn to listen to what your body is telling you. You may have spent much of your life in body-avoidance, so you'll have to train yourself to tune in to body messages.

Here's a case in point. Maybe you're a sweet-craver. Most overweights are. Learn to anticipate problems and to substitute. Instead of nutrient-poor refined sugars and starches, try some "real food" such as fruit or crunchy vegetables high in natural sugars. They keep your blood sugar levels up so you don't feel that "crash" between meals. You can make anything work if you want to, can't you?

What have you done right today? You are keeping an ear tuned to what your body tells you. Because you have taken responsibility for your health, you want to learn how food works for you and what to do when it doesn't.

Today's Action Plan: I will eat energy foods that help me control weight. I accept responsibility for what I eat.

Starving vs. Exercise

Diet. Exercise. Attitude.
Don't pick one — pick them all.
Editors of *Executive Fitness Newsletter*

Exercise is an essential tool for weight control. In the past, you may have been among those who thought they could just cut back on calories, and skip all the sweating. Sorry. Calorie-cutting is no alternative to physical activity. No one's saying that exercise is *more* important than diet; but we know it's an equal partner. Now that you're feeling lighter and healthier, you're better able to exercise, aren't you?

You may have lost weight fast on low-calorie diets without exercise. But let's look at that weight loss. The first thing that happens with calorie restriction alone is that your body uses its glycogen (stored sugar). When you reduce calories you use your stored energy to run your body. When one pound of glycogen goes, as much as four pounds of water exit with it, not fat, but water. This shows up as your instant weight loss. Next goes protein from muscle tissue. But it's muscle that you want to keep, if you intend to look better. No wonder you feel fatigued and become less active, which further slows down fat loss. Low-calorie diets alone won't help you build a new LifeWay. You're getting the picture, aren't you?

What have you done right today? You recognized the potential harm in the extra-low calorie, no-exercise approach to weight loss. You have decided not to throw this book across the room, but to read on.

Today's Action Plan: I will eat and exercise for health. I will keep an open mind to the idea of exercise.

Exercise vs. Fat

Dieting . . . removes . . . fat only under the most severe
prison camp circumstances. A well-exercised body seems
to respond more quickly and with less muscle loss . . .
Covert Bailey

It takes several weeks before the body begins to shed fat
on a restricted-calorie diet with no exercise. "It may take
longer," you think, "but this way I won't have to
exercise at all." Not true! More than twice the calories
are stored in a pound of fat than are stored in either a
pound of protein or sugar; losing the fat is a much
slower process by diet alone. (So the diet that rewarded
you with a five-pound loss per week in the beginning
now only gives a one-pound-per-week loss of body fat.
You're wondering why, aren't you?)

Something is happening that you can blame on ances-
tral conditioning. Human fat cells have learned to reduce
their activity in response to famine. So if you go on
eating less (after all the glycogen and muscle protein is
gone), your fat cells will protect themselves by actually
burning off much more slowly. As a matter of fact, your
basal metabolism (the rate calories burn in your body)
may slow to almost half its former rate. At this point, if
you go off your diet and begin to overeat, you'll regain
weight faster than you lost it.

You can beat the old lose-gain cycle. There's one way
— exercise. It will speed up your metabolism and your
fat tissue will once again begin to vanish. You've really
got the answer this time, haven't you?

What have you done right today? You learned how
your body handles calories. You discovered that exercise
and diet are perfect partners. You're getting very smart!

**Today's Action Plan: I will continue to exercise so I
can lose weight more successfully than ever before. I will
not reject the idea of making exercise a habit.**

March 22

Exercise to Thinness

Over many thousands of years, since before the dawn of civilization, our bodies have been geared to and sustained by habitual and extensive physical activity.
Dr. Kenneth H. Cooper

The last two days you learned about the frustration of dieting *without* exercise. Now for the good news — the joy of dieting *with* exercise. Nature built into your body a wonderful protective device. Here's how it works: calorie intake and expenditure automatically adjust to maintain a natural body weight, but only if you are active. When prehistoric people were evolving, they had to be in shape and ready to run from danger. Today you don't need to flee from saber-toothed tigers, but from an over-abundance of food and leisure. You are becoming more convinced that exercise is what's missing from your life, aren't you?

Here's what exercise promises to every overweight: If you exercise reasonably vigorously your body will continue to burn calories for fifteen hours at a higher rate than it would have without exercise. It's like tuning your car's engine to idle faster — you burn more fuel.

If your metabolism is on the slow side (and it is, if you're an overweight who's been on and off many diets), regular exercise can boost your metabolism from 20 to 30 percent. That translates into a much lower weight for you. You be the mathematician. How much would 20 to 30 percent faster burning of calories mean to you in pounds?

What have you done right today? You have learned what exercise can do for your body. You have determined that exercise gives you a calorie-burning bonus.

Today's Action Plan: I will raise my metabolism twice today. I will be body-aware.

Exercise to Burn Calories

*Losing weight was never my problem — I've lost a
zillion pounds. But the only way I ever kept it off was
putting my body into action.*

Georgia Alban

Now that you're not resisting the idea of exercise quite so
much, let's see how you can use it to enhance the high-
energy life you're aiming for. First, accept that you'll lose
weight faster and be healthier if you exercise. Second,
accept the fact that dieters can help control weight with
regular physical exercise. Do you accept these two ideas?
Say YES, out loud.

There are a few tricks to exercise that you should
know. It is best to split your exercise into two periods,
one at the start and the other at the end of the day. You
don't have to run a marathon or climb the Matterhorn
— just twenty minutes of brisk walking will do it.

If you should slip off your diet plan don't sit and
berate yourself. Exercise will get rid of those excess
calories, producing body heat which literally burns up
calories.

Try alternating three aerobic activities, like bicycling,
walking, and jogging (or any other combination) so you
won't get bored repeating the same activity each day.
You will do that, won't you?

What have you done right today? You have decided
to accept physical activity as a faster and healthier way
to the thin life.

**Today's Action Plan: I will make exercise as much a
part of my daily routine as combing my hair. I will take
charge of my body.**

Twenty-five Hour Day

*The greatest freedom you have is the freedom to disci-
pline yourself.*

Bernard M. Baruch

A winner's life has a certain rhythm, a discipline. A
winner takes everyday things in stride; handles daily
details routinely. When you do this, there is much more
time to maneuver creatively. You will find that establish-
ing a routine for the details of your days means you
won't have to make endless decisions about unimportant
things. As soon as you get the "everydayness" out of the
way, your life becomes unbelievably free. Having a
disciplined routine squeezes an extra hour from every
day. You can use those extra hours for fun, can't you?

Winners get up about the same time every day, eat at
the same times, and do all they have to do in about the
same number of hours so that they can get proper rest.
Into their day they have programmed exercise, right-
eating, and time for themselves. They know what they're
supposed to do every day, *and they do it.* They leave
time to think and plan for the future. They have time for
relaxation and fun, and time for family and friends.

Does that sound boring? Think about it. If you are
overeating or you remember when you did, what was
your day like? Sick, desperate, tired. You longed for
some structure in your life, whether you called it that or
not. You never want days without structure again, do
you?

What have you done right today? You have decided
that the structure of a high-energy, achieving life is what
you want. You need never go back to overeating again.
And that's a promise.

Today's Action Plan: I will enjoy the freedom of
discipline. I will seek it in everyday life.

You Can Do It

*It is in men as in soils, where sometimes there is a vein
of gold, which the owner knows not of.*
Jonathan Swift

Do you believe you can do everything you have to do,
and ninety-nine percent of what you want to do? Say
YES. For too long you listened to a negative litany in
your head that went: "I can't do that. I have no training/
talent/money." Or even worse, "I'm just not smart
enough." Nonsense! The average human being can
achieve practically anything, and you're above average.
You gave up being average the minute you picked up
this book. You're through with negative mindtalk, aren't
you?

Out with that destructive talk. Don't tell yourself that
you've tried every diet, every exercise, every doctor, and
there's no way out of overeating. This plants a powerful,
destructive thought in your head. In effect, you've closed
your mind to new ideas and told yourself there's no hope
for you. Don't do that!

Every day tell yourself that you're ready to adopt new
ideas. Tell others that change is a challenge for you. Day
by day, break down your old negativity and replace it
with a positive, dynamic new self-image. Soon you'll
begin to think of yourself as open-minded, quick to
master new information, new ways. Your mind, instead
of being blocked, will begin to filter what you see and
hear through the outline of your needs and wants. Do
you want such an open mind? Say YES.

What have you done right today? You have declared
that you are attracted to new ideas, so that new ideas
will be attracted to you.

Today's Action Plan: I will build a new helpful self-
image. I will open my mind to the world.

Now Is the Time

*To every thing there is a season, and a time to every
purpose under the heaven.*

Ecclesiastes 3:1

This is your season, your day to start becoming the
person you want to be. Beginning today will end an old
conflict that raged inside you, a conflict caused by your
fight against your dreams of what you could become.
This very second is the time to shift from dependency, to
stop relying on food for comfort and leaning on other
people to tell you who you are. It's time to be an
independent, self-reliant adult. You agree with that, don't
you?

Tell yourself that you have a solution to the problem
of overeating which is well within your ability to
achieve. You are the only boss on the job. On your
journey to high-energy wellness, you will be busy. The
old habit of overeating takes constant supervision to
control, but now you have the managerial ability to
handle this challenge.

Remember, your old habit of overeating to soothe
your day, solve your problems, and make you feel better
about yourself, never worked. When you overate, your
day was likely to be a shambles, your problems were
overwhelming, and your self-esteem was at zero. But this
is your season. You have let go of overeating as a
solution to living problems. Reach out into the winner's
future, won't you?

What have you done right today? You know your
time has come to set goals and go after them. You are
confident that you have enormous reserves of untapped
power, and you're going to start using them. Do it.

**Today's Action Plan: I will make today the season of
my beginning. I will let go of overeating and march
ahead to a winner's future.**

March 27

Lady Luck

The harder I work, the luckier I get.
Anonymous

Think about that: the harder you work, the luckier you'll be; *you make your own luck.* Too many people sit back and wait for luck to knock at their door — they see Lady Luck as a mother substitute. Luck doesn't work like that. Luck is a change that you have to recognize and be ready for; it's all around you; you pass it every day without seeing it, because you haven't trained yourself to see it. How often do you think you may have passed luck without knowing it?

The more you work at self-understanding, the more you take Action on what you learn, then the more ready you will be for luck when it comes your way. Take, for example, an exciting idea about nutrition you might pick up by studying how bodies work. By using a winner's curious mind to learn the way your body works, this new idea will mean something special to you. You won't miss it. You'll grasp the brass ring. How "lucky" you'll be!

Work hard at the changes you are making in your life. Learn and study and think. You'll get lucky. That's a promise. Believe that, won't you?

What have you done right today? You've seen that luck isn't something you fall into, but something you prepare yourself to recognize. That's an important idea. Don't forget it.

Today's Action Plan: I will prepare myself so that I can take advantage of every opportunity. I will work hard so that Lady Luck will become a frequent visitor.

March 28

Do You Have Binge Foods?

*I can't drink a little, therefore I never touch it. Absti-
nence is as easy to me as temperance would be difficult.*
Samuel Johnson

Many of us have reactions to foods we can't control,
foods we are absolutely addicted to. The first bite leads
to countless others, beyond the point of hunger, beyond
the point of craving. We are helpless to stop. A binge
food can be almost anything. One woman at a diet
group meeting needed a "bologna fix" periodically
through her day. But most binge foods are sweet, gooey
confections that we use as constant rewards. If you have
a binge food, whatever it is, you may have to give it up
entirely. Before you yell "NO," read to the bottom of the
page, will you?

*Giving up binge foods is easier than struggling con-
stantly to control them.* You know your own binge
foods, you're thinking about them right now. One bite is
too much and a whole box/batch/bowl isn't enough.
Right? Do you have any idea how much energy you use
trying to control your desire for and consumption of
these foods, energy you could be spending to get a thin
body? There's no winning with binge foods. Whatever
the cause, sugar craving, memories of mommy, it's too
powerful to control while you're feeding your habit.

Don't try to eat just one. It takes all your energy to
stop, and you can't do it. Isn't that right? Will you get
rid of your binge foods now, and play the game to win?
Please, say YES.

What have you done right today? You have discovered that it is much easier to get rid of binge foods than
to struggle with them in your eating plan.

**Today's Action Plan: I will get rid of my binge foods.
I will not allow any food to keep me from greatness.**

You'd Rather Fly

*One can never consent to creep when one feels the
impulse to soar.*

Helen Keller

You were born to fly, to soar high above the ordinary
and average. How long have you been tied to the
ground by your compulsion to overeat? Too long! If
you're creeping instead of flying, the conflict of not
doing what you know you can is wrecking your life.
That's true, isn't it?

Make a deep commitment to earn a thinner body, and
the wonderful things that overweight has stopped you
from achieving. Start now.

A funny thing about commitment, it makes you feel
better instantly. Food never did that for you; instead,
overeating always made you feel worse about yourself.

You don't get something for nothing; there's a fee for
admission into the achieving life. You pay by working
on self-understanding, staying on a weight-losing eating
plan, and exercising regularly. Does that sound like a lot
of work? Not when you're building the health and self-
confidence you want. Not when you compare it with
what you get back. Best of all, you'll be in charge of
your own life.

If you make the commitment and put your plan into
Action, you can soar for the rest of your days. You
deserve that, don't you?

What have you done right today? You took charge of
your own wellness today. You know there's a price to
pay, but that the price is nothing compared to the pain
of overeating. Be well, right now.

Today's Action Plan: I will put my desire for a well,
thin body into Action. I will soar instead of creep.

Your Great Friend Adversity

*Adversity has the effect of eliciting talents which, in
prosperous circumstances, would have lain dormant.*
                                                    Horace

Do you know how lucky you are? You have a curable
problem. You can do something about your overeating,
right now, today. More than that, you're lucky because
the pain of being overweight in a society that makes a
cult of thinness has made you stronger than steel. You
hadn't thought of that, had you?

Think about it. If you didn't have some steel in you,
you wouldn't be the curious and searching person that
you are. You are constantly seeking alternative paths to
your goals. Many people resist change and act out their
negative, destructive habits their whole life long. Not
you. You are open to new ideas because you want a life
that works.

You may have your faults — everyone does — but a
lack of courage isn't one of them. No matter how many
times you tried to stop overeating and failed in the past,
you have the courage to try again. That makes you
special.

Every day you uncover talents you never dreamed
you had because you keep on trying no matter what
adversity you face. Remember that the next time you are
self-critical. Yes, remember that.

What have you done right today? You have recognized that adversity, rather than destroying you, gave
you strength and persistence. Can you see how this
makes you one of the special people? Say YES.

Today's Action Plan: I will not begrudge the pain I've
suffered because it uncovered talents I didn't know I had.
I will continue to play life to win no matter what.

Under the Circumstances

In the fell clutch of circumstance . . .
William Ernest Henley

Without goals that are specifically stated and worked for, overeaters float along without anchors. Circumstances control us. Any event, good or bad, can be an excuse to overeat. We eat to celebrate; we eat to grieve. Don't you agree that happens?

We overeaters repeatedly tell how we ate in response to almost every conceivable emotional circumstance. We say, "When I was happy I ate to celebrate. When I was sad I ate to quiet the anguish. And I ate for every feeling in between, because overeating was the only response I had to what happened to me."

Set goals in all areas of your life and make them harmonize with your goal to lose your excess weight and maintain it. Winners set goals each day, which they constantly review and fine tune. Make your goals specific. Tell yourself the number of pounds you want to lose; decide what specific job you want with your company; list the actual improvement you want in your life. Write your goals so that you can *see* them. You can do that, can't you?

What have you done right today? You discovered that when you stay on your right-eating plan, you control circumstances, they don't control you. Feel your emotions instead of feeding them, and you've placed yourself solidly in charge of your life.

Today's Action Plan: I will take charge of the circumstances of my life. Whatever they are, I will make them better by abstaining from overeating.

The Worst Vulgarity

*. . . habitual vulgarity . . . in an individual . . . is
extraordinarily unhealthy, because it mocks the things of
the spirit, and slowly squeezes out all serious thought, all
fruitful discourse and all genuine sentiment.*
Bryan F. Griffin

Would you make a public joke about someone's height,
nose, ears? Of course not. It would be unkind, even
vulgar, wouldn't it?

Although Griffin's quotation refers to the four-letter
kind of vulgarity, his assessment holds especially true for
those overweights who abuse *themselves* publicly. "Vulgarity" also applies to the jolly fat victim making himself
the butt of his own fat-jokes. "I'm shade in the summer
and heat in the winter," announced one woman in front
of her friends. "Better guard your good chairs," guffawed
an overweight man at a party. "I'm gonna kill 'em!"

We really don't want people to believe us, but too
often they do. When we run into the same group, some
wandering wit will yell, "Hey, Blobbo, how ya' doing?"

The Good Sport Syndrome — an effort to show
people we really don't care about our weight by drawing
comic attention to ourselves — is the worst vulgarity
that can come out of our mouths. It says to others that
we see ourselves as clowns, and don't take ourselves
seriously.

But the new you will never try to make yourself
popular at the expense of your dignity. Nevermore.
From this day forward, you're going to respect yourself,
isn't that right?

What have you done right today? You have learned
that if you don't respect your own dignity, no one else
will.

**Today's Action Plan: I will not be a jolly fat victim. I
will respect myself, within myself, and before other
people.**

Living Life

Life is the thing that really happens to us while we are making other plans.

Anonymous

Overeaters have been diagnosed as having grandiose personalities. We make big plans. We start the race with a burst of speed. What happens? We have a little slip, something doesn't go the way we'd planned, some special person doesn't read the script the way we wrote it, and — wham! — to heck with it. We chuck it all — diet, plans, good intentions. You know people who are great starters, but never finish the race, don't you?

There are two ways you can live. The first begins with overeating and trying to manipulate people to gain their approval; it ends in overweight and loneliness.

The second way begins with abstinence from overeating, with a desire for an independent, high-energy life; it ends in fulfillment. The choice, as always, is yours.

Ask yourself two questions. Have you made plans for your life? As a result of these plans, has your life improved? If you answered both questions negatively, life is just happening to you, and you don't seem to have much to say about it.

Look inside yourself, decide what you want, and begin to work for it; put your wants into Action. Your life will agree with your plans, and you'll move in the direction you want to go.

What have you done right today? You have decided not to let life pass you by. You compared two ways you could live your life and you chose the one that leads to your happiness.

Today's Action Plan: I will not allow life just to happen to me. I will make plans and put them into Action.

Face It

*You don't get a second chance to make
a first impression.*

Vidal Sassoon

Psychologists tell us the face is the part of the body which best reflects emotions. All your life you've been chided — by mother, by teacher, by friends — to "put on a happy face." Take that advice today, not so much because your smile might please others, but because it is important to you. You are willing to learn more about that idea, aren't you?

Some overeaters think their faces are only for others to see, but your face also communicates all sorts of messages to *you.* If you are typical of most overweight people, you don't want to look at your body in the mirror, but you don't hesitate to look at your face. How do you communicate with that face?

Do you put on a big smile for others, and a big frown for yourself? Are you a man who combs his hair and shaves — for others? Are you a woman who plucks her eyebrows and puts on eye shadow — for others? Then, do you give yourself a scowl?

Choose to send a you-deserve-a-good-day message when you give yourself the first impression of the morning. Turn on a friendly face. Drop the sneer and choose the cheer. Start off the day really liking yourself. Try it, won't you? Make a YES decision, right now.

What have you done right today? You have learned the importance of putting on your best, friendliest, least critical face — for yourself. Isn't that better?

Today's Action Plan: I will give myself positive messages in my mirror. I will make a good first impression — on me!

April 4

After Exercise

I won't tell you that getting used to daily exercise is a bed of roses, but remember, it's your muscles that burn the vast majority of your calories, and even the best diets combined with the most potent vitamins will never tune up your muscles the way good exercise will.

Covert Bailey

Most exercise-to-expend-calories charts are half-right; they give only part of the story. If you go by the charts, exercise hardly seems worth the trouble. Jog twenty minutes and lose 180 calories — about what you get in a glass of milk. Forget it! Have you said that before?

But calorie-loss isn't the greatest benefit of exercise. Studies have shown that exercise changes your body's metabolic rate, and increases calorie-burn long after you stop exercising. Physically fit people who exercise daily burn more calories than sedentary people — even when they're asleep.

Exercise for the overweight is probably more frustrating than dieting ever was, because results are slow. Be patient. Although the stored fat won't melt overnight, it will gradually be replaced by muscle and taut skin.

Your goal need not be the Olympics, but it's reasonable to expect your body to firm so that you're able to walk or climb stairs without puffing and turning red in the face. So start exercising for fitness. You need stamina for the high-energy life you're leading, don't you?

What have you done right today? You have acknowledged the importance of physical exercise in your winning program. You know that with exercise your body will burn rather than store fat. That's what you want.

Today's Action Plan: I will exercise my body for physical and emotional satisfaction. I will get the most out of my body today.

April 5

Dreams

If you want your dreams to come true, don't sleep.
                                                    Yiddish Proverb

Are you a dreamer? Do you dream of waking up thin some morning? Nothing wrong with that. Go ahead and dream, dream great dreams, but don't wait passively for them to come true. Make them come true. You'd like to do that, wouldn't you?

Believe your dreams: what you can dream, you can believe; what you can believe, you can achieve.

A thin body and a winning life are your goals. You can dream of such a happy future, but first cast aside all past failures. You will be free, as if by magic, when you let go of old regrets, recriminations, and excuses. It's the only way. You can't travel into a positive tomorrow with yesterday's negative baggage.

Tell someone about this happy dream. The more you hear yourself say it, the more you will believe. It was never dreaming you feared — you were only afraid of failing. That fear grew until it stifled all belief, until the only dreams your mind could conceive were puny, stunted things. Dream great dreams, and make them come true, won't you?

What have you done right today? You have decided not to stifle your great dreams. You know that by believing in your dreams, wonderful things will happen.

Today's Action Plan: I will unlock my dream power. I will dream dreams of a high-energy life and make them come true.

April 6

A Tool Kit for Action

If the only tool you have is a hammer, you tend to see every problem as a nail.
Abraham Maslow

When you overate, you were angry with yourself, you were, as the AA saying goes, "sick and tired of feeling sick and tired." You tended to illuminate all your problems with the lamp of your anger. Every problem was a nail, and your only response was to hammer on it. You'd like a more versatile tool kit than that, wouldn't you?

The high-energy life will require a wide array of attitudes (tools). Problems will test you, but don't let them arrest you. Pull one of the MindSteps from your repair kit and start to work. You can't be stopped if you have the tools to make things right. With a positive, constructive attitude, you will find solutions for obstacles. With anger as your only tool, you will fail to find solutions. Without solutions, you may give up — the biggest mistake of all.

If your problem doesn't respond to attitude, reason, or MindSteps, then you know *you* are probably your problem.

Don't get angry, get going. Say YES, won't you?

What have you done right today? You have learned that if you have an insoluble problem, the problem is usually you. You stopped hammering on your problems, and learned to work through them. Now, you've hit it on the head!

Today's Action Plan: Instead of anger, I will use the power of my mind. I will enlarge my kit of Action tools.

Caring

*Friend: One who knows all about you and loves you
just the same.*

Elbert Hubbard

Some overeaters pull away from other people fearing
rejection. Theirs is a special loneliness because they have
bought society's fat stereotype and think of themselves as
passive, people to whom things are done, rather than
people who do things. Have you protected yourself from
prejudice, and paid the price in loneliness?

Hold it! Don't accept the destructive fat stereotype. It's
a false image and inconsistent with the winner emerging
from within you. Don't ever buy it. Not ever!

But do accept people who want to be your friends,
people who can see you as you really are. Don't let your
fear of rejection drive others away before you discover
their genuine feelings.

If you feel lonely, be a friend. Read the third Action
MindStep: **Radiate warmth.** Show others that you can
care. Caring people are magnets, drawing others to
them. Try being a friend today, won't you? Say YES.

What have you done right today? You rejected the
idea that we overweights aren't worth knowing. To earn
friendship, you have learned you must be a friend. It's a
risk, but that's better than being lonely. Good for you.

**Today's Action Plan: I will get rid of my stereotypical
fat image. When I'm lonely, I will be a friend to myself
and to others.**

April 8

Why You're Reading this Book

It is not necessary to hope in order to undertake, nor to succeed in order to persevere.

Blaise Pascal

You're holding this book on purpose. You know you need help, and you're searching for a way out of your overeating problem. Your choice of this book reveals that your helplessness and hopelessness have been burned away by your flame of hope. Reading these words proves it. That's true, isn't it?

Your false starts are past. You've discovered the right course of Action. Don't berate yourself because it took you so long to reach this day. A winner tries many methods before self-motivation and Action lead to victory.

When you begin to *do*, instead of waiting for others to do *to* you, you take control of your direction. You move forward, like a winner. There may be temporary adjustments along the way, but you will continue your weight control program. Your determination to persevere feels good, doesn't it?

What have you done right today? You have seen that while you may have tried to hide in inaction to protect yourself from another disappointment, a flame of hope still burns in you.

Today's Action Plan: I will cherish the bright flame of hope. I will be a victor, not a victim.

Read this, if You Can't Stick to Exercising

The stock approach to the fat person is to start him on a diet as the first order of business and to worry about the rest later, and of course, "later" never really comes.
Dr. William Bennett

Have you repeatedly started a regular exercise regimen, but for some reason couldn't stick to it? If so, you may have subconsciously thought of yourself as an invalid, someone who is incapable of physical exercise. How could this be?

Western medicine has traditionally seen overweight as an overeating problem with a reducing diet as its cure. Since most diet-only programs are unsuccessful, other kinds of health care such as exercise and attitude changes never seem to get started. Most often, overweights are seen as chronic patient failures and, as such, invalids.

What do you expect from invalids? Unfortunate as the stereotype may be, we perceive invalids as those who restrict their activities and remove themselves from circulation. Even the word "invalid" means without worth.

Do you think you might have the idea that you are an invalid? Could this be the real reason you have trouble seeing yourself as a physical person? Think about it, won't you?

What have you done right today? You discovered one reason you might have trouble perceiving yourself as a physical person. You also saw that understanding is the basis for Action.

Today's Action Plan: I will prove that I am not an invalid. I will discover the active person within me.

April 10

The Action Habit

Actions speak louder than words.

Old saying

Action is character. You may argue that character is a combination of personality traits, good and bad. But you must agree that people are what they do — not what they say. A man with a particular sense of humor sees things slightly askew and comments wryly. A woman with a reputation for honesty tells the truth. Without their Actions, people are blanks. Only through acts do we know ourselves and others. Don't you agree?

Character isn't set in concrete, no matter how old your habits are — like overeating, eating the wrong foods, and avoiding physical activity. Your habits can be changed. Don't try to fight or bend them (that's like one hand wrestling the other); change negative actions by replacing them with positive new actions and habits.

What you do is what you are. Yesterday's wrongs are gone, replaced by today's Action. Don't feel you are forever mired in your past actions. You can let them go. Today you can and will do things that will change your character. Say YES, won't you?

What have you done right today? You see how you can change your character by doing what you want to become. You see that Action leads directly to the thinner, high-energy, achieving life you want. Think about it. It really does make sense.

Today's Action Plan: I will do the things it takes to become who I want to be. I will not wrestle with old behavior, but simply change it, replace it with something new.

April 11

Break Out of the Fat Trap

*I was always the one the family came to when something
had to be done. "Jerri can do it" was a family joke.
That's why I blamed everything but me for being fat. It
was my way of denying that I had a need I couldn't fill.*
                                                    Jerri Hannah

Anyone who sincerely wants to get out of the fat trap
can escape by increasing self-understanding. Remember
the difference between self-awareness and self-understanding? Self-awareness recognizes feelings; self-understanding does something about them. Self-awareness
accepts things as they are; self-understanding realizes that
change is possible and develops a plan for change. But
before you can have self-understanding, you have to get
rid of all the lies you believe — like your supposed
inability to lose weight permanently. You can see that,
can't you?

We overeaters lie to ourselves. As self-deceivers, we
deny the reality of what we're doing to our lives; we say,
"I'm not overeating — fat runs in my family." We look
for scapegoats by blaming others for our overweight. We
search for magic answers. We say we're finished with
trying, pretending not to care. But when the pain breaks
through, reality is there staring us in the face.

Embrace reality. Self-deception feeds on fresh lies
every day; self-understanding is nurtured by what is real
and true. When you stop lying to yourself about who
you are and what you want, self-deception will vanish
from the scene. Trust that, won't you?

What have you done right today? You made a YES
decision to face your life as it is, without pretense. You
see that self-understanding and self-deception can't coex-
ist and you're going to be honest with yourself.

**Today's Action Plan: I will tell myself the truth. I'll
embrace reality so my Actions take me where I want to
go.**

April 12

Try Again, Now that You've Changed

We are new every day.
Irene Claremont de Castillego

Sometimes we get a mindset about our behavior. We change, but don't realize we've changed, so we continue to act in old, inappropriate ways. Shyness, particularly if carried over from childhood, is one of the traits we often keep. Have you tested yourself lately for any such inhibiting mindsets?

A capable government engineer's job required him to attend meetings. During meetings he hid in a corner, trying to be invisible. When the meeting ended he hurried away, for fear that someone would call on him to speak. Oddly, he was self-assured at other times. When asked about why he never contributed in meetings, he said, "I've been shy in groups since I was a boy." Hearing this, a new man in the department laughed and said, "You, shy? Why, you're the most competent man here."

During the next meeting, the engineer voluntarily explained a complicated plan without a stumble. The only difference was his Action. He'd stopped being shy long ago, he just hadn't discovered it; his shyness was a habit of thinking, not a fact. Do you have some habitual behavior that makes you say: "Oh, no. I can't. I'm too shy (or too old, or too fat)." How long has it been since you checked?

What have you done right today? You have seen that it is easy to keep fixed thinking that no longer applies to you.

Today's Action Plan: I will do what I've convinced myself I couldn't do. I will take the first opportunity to try my wings.

April 13

It's No Sin

Eating has become the last bona fide sin.
Ellen Goodman

Overweight isn't immoral; thinness isn't moral. Good and bad have nothing at all to do with overeating. When you finally understand this, you'll be able to put recrimination behind you. You believe this, don't you?

As an overweight, you must withstand our culture's thin-is-in attitudes of blame, loathing, and mockery. You don't have to cooperate by believing this negative image. As Action MindStep number ten says: **Reject rejection firmly and totally** — from others and from yourself.

Every day you are building a dynamic image of yourself. Therefore, don't predict your own failure, don't laugh at your goals, don't allow anyone to deter you from your new life. Now *you* are in charge.

You've made a YES decision about your life. Since that commitment you have handled rejection by rejecting it and tossing out self-doubt. You adore your new positive attitudes, don't you? Say YES. Then say it again.

What have you done right today? You have come to understand that overweight is not a moral problem, but one of attitude, right-eating, and exercise.

Today's Action Plan: I will not be defined by my weight. I will not think of myself as a sinner, but as someone with a health problem that I'm doing something about.

April 14

Afraid of Diet Success?

You know not how to live in clover.
Menander

You learned to live with overeating. You managed to accomodate the demands of an overeating life. Bad as your life was when you ate compulsively — when food, not you, was in charge — at least the routine was familiar: binge, regret, diet, slip, binge — you know the familiar routine. That destructive cycle was so much a part of your daily existence that you couldn't imagine any other. You even feared diet success because it was unknown. You recognize this, don't you?

Your old life was built around the false joy of overeating. Now that you've found a dynamic new LifeWay, you've lost the imagined pleasure of overeating, but you've also rid yourself of pounds and pain. Forget the old ways; food is no longer at the center of your life. Success is your new center. Think about success in a constructive way. It's important.

Think of what positive things you can do to fill the huge vacuum left now that food is no longer your way of life. Winners who *get rid* of pounds and pain can fill up with success.

Don't regret your change. Don't fear diet success. Welcome it. You can cope with a creative, constructive life. You can learn to live with success, can't you?

What have you done right today? You acknowledged that any fear of diet success is really a thinking problem. You know that the pain of overeating is too high a price to pay for maintaining familiar old patterns. You want the real joy and rewards of a full, in-control life and a thinner you.

Today's Action Plan: I will know that doing without food is not deprivation, but privilege. I will find ways to fill any emptiness with my new winner's attitude.

Which Are You?

People can be divided into three groups: those who make things happen, those who watch things happen — and those who wonder what happened.
Yiddish Proverb

Winners dare. They dare to make their dreams become reality; they have the audacity to go into Action and get what they want. When are you going to make your thoughts become the things you want? The answer is: immediately. You have this ability. Believe it, won't you?

Thinness is a natural desire; it is perfectly natural to want it. Go ahead. Take the time to nurture this desire. Visualize it. Don't be distracted. Give all of your attention to your dream. Commit yourself to achieving the body you want. Yes, there is an element of risk, but without risk there can be no success. Remember you're playing to win. Convince yourself that you can succeed.

Which of the three groups in the proverb do you want to belong to? Do you want forever to watch the parade go by? Do you want to be out of control and wonder what happened? Or do you want to make things happen?

You are a person who makes things happen. You can succeed, if you invest in yourself. Take a MindStep every day, won't you?

What have you done right today? You decided which group you want to belong to and dared to desire thinness. This is true, so say YES.

Today's Action Plan: I will make things happen. I will begin now.

April 16

Getting Even

Success is the best revenge.

French Proverb

If you were an overweight child, you may be haunted by childhood memories of school yard bullies. As an overweight adolescent, you remember being excluded from the fun of teen years. Now, as an overweight adult, you may face discrimination on the job and ridicule by society. You have a right to be angry if you've been recognized only as a weight, not a person. But don't get mad, get success. That's the best way to put ugly memories to rest. Think about it, won't you?

You're not a weight, you're an important human being. You have made thinness a goal because you want a high-energy, in-control life. You want to feel great, look wonderful in your clothes, and deal with your weight problem successfully so that you can get on with your life. And there's more to life, so much more than you ever dreamed there would be. You have made a YES decision. You have decided to join the winner's circle and put past hurts behind you. Isn't that right?

What have you done right today? You have decided that the way to erase ugly memories is to fill the rest of your life with achievement. And you'll do it, too.

Today's Action Plan: I will lose weight because I want to get more out of life. After all the laughter and cruelties, I will achieve a unique place in this world.

Less Is More

People have to be informed and more aware of nutrients in foods, so that they can make intelligent individual choices.

Dr. Kathleen Zolber

There are many books on good nutrition. Get one and read it to learn what the nutritional needs are of your eating and exercise plan. This is up to you. The information is available. Set a goal to learn about your own food needs. Plan to cut back on sugar, fat, and salt in your nutrition program. Won't you give such a program careful thought?

Abusing these three substances can cause problems like heart disease and tooth decay, as well as retard weight loss and maintenance.

- Limit fat by reducing dairy foods, saturated oils, and red meat.
- Limit salt by adding only small amounts for cooking and none at the table. Reduce or eliminate salty snack foods.
- Limit refined sugar by completely eliminating or drastically reducing sweets. (You know what these are.)

You already know which of these foods need to be reduced or eliminated from your diet. What you haven't done is put your knowledge into Action. By limiting fat, salt, and sugar, you'll meet an important nutritional goal. Isn't that right?

What have you done right today? You have decided to learn more about nutrition so you can make wise food selections. As you reduce the negative effects of food each day, you increase food's positive uses. Not a bad day's work.

Today's Action Plan: I will reduce or eliminate salt, fat, and sugar. I will say YES to good nutrition.

April 18

A Pound of Flesh

The law of life is that when growth ceases, decay and decline begin.

Henry Clay Lindgren

When it comes to demanding attitudes about extracting that extra "pound of flesh" (in this case, our own), we overeaters can outdo Shakespeare's Shylock. Do you have a blaming, prejudicial attitude toward your weight? That's a self-hateful way to live. If you want to help yourself make your life work better, you can't be your own worst enemy. Stop the self-blame. Concentrate on self-help, won't you?

Don't dwell on negatives. Take inventory of the positive things about you. Your tenacious hold on hope shows that there is something special about you. There are many marvelous qualities buried under your negative self-image. Take them out, look at them, and say, "I'm a nice person. I don't have any reason to be ashamed." Say that. Out loud. It doesn't matter if someone over-hears; people already know your good qualities. You're the one who needs to be convinced.

Don't harass yourself. The next time you bad-mouth yourself, stop and point to one of your positive qualities instead. Do it. You weren't embarrassed when you said unkind things about yourself, so don't be embarrassed to say nice things. That's fair, isn't it? Say YES.

What have you done right today? You have acknowledged that you often treat yourself worse than you would allow anyone else to treat you. You have decided not to harass yourself any longer.

Today's Action Plan: From now on, I will replace my own tough demand to extract my pound of flesh with my positive program of self-understanding, diet and exercise. I will be fair to myself.

A Powerful Motivator

recognition: an acknowledgement
Webster's Unabridged Dictionary

A motivator is something people respond to in a gut-level way. Powerful motivators drive us to our goals. One of the most powerful of all motivators is recognition. You'd like to know how to get recognition, wouldn't you?

It's simple. First you have to achieve, and to achieve, you act.

Compulsive personalities — the kind many overeaters have — seem to demand more approval from the world than the world is willing to give. We manipulate; please this one and that one to make them say that we're important to them. And we may be successful praise-wheedlers for a time, but those negative inner voices keep telling us how unworthy we are.

You're absolutely right to want recognition, but no one can hand it to you. Only babies are recognized for just being here — adults have to earn it. Here's the formula again: Action equals achievement equals recognition. That creates a wonderful feeling of security and satisfaction. It feels great, doesn't it? No doubt about it.

What have you done right today? Now you know the right way to earn the acknowledgment you've always wanted. Remember the formula, and get it!

Today's Action Plan: I will seek recognition through achievement. I will aim for goals which demand achievement.

Be Prepared to Walk Alone

Alone, alone, all, all alone
Alone on a wide wide sea!
                    Samuel Taylor Coleridge

You'll never be as alone as the ancient mariner, but if you make a commitment to high performance, real achievement, you'll have to accept the consequences of that commitment.

Perhaps you won't be as available to others as in the past. You may even have to say no when you are asked to do something that might jeopardize your recovery. Here's a simple case in point: You are asked to pick up ice cream on your way home. Ice cream is a food you avoid. Therefore you have to say no until you are stronger. You see the point, don't you?

Ultimately you have to stand alone. You have friends, family, co-weight-losers, co-workers — many people who wish you well — but when you stand toe-to-toe, slugging it out with temptation, you fight alone. There are times when others can help, and that's wonderful. But when no one can help you but yourself, you have to be ready.

It's not selfish to take care of yourself. How much were you able to do for others when you were overeating? Now that you are committed to health goals you have energy for others that you didn't have before. But you'll have to say no, when you must, to protect your commitment. You can stand alone when you must, can't you? Say YES.

What have you done right today? You have seen that you must put personal commitment to achievement before pleasing people. You do this so that you can be of real use to yourself and ultimately to others.

Today's Action Plan: I will stand alone to protect my commitment when I must. I will resolve not to jeopardize my recovery from overeating.

April 21

Your Own Way

They are able because they think they are able.

Virgil

One way to rid yourself of a hurtful compulsion is to fill your mind with a helpful one. Overeating is a hurtful compulsion. Freedom from overeating can be a helpful compulsion. Have you ever considered the possibility of positive compulsion?

Getting rid of the compulsion to overeat is not easy. But overeating causes you so much pain and discomfort, and you want to rid yourself of the pain, to gain self-control. Self-control is another name for freedom from food.

You have an idea of what you should be doing. When you refuse to acknowledge that idea, when you turn your back on your wants and try to drown them in food, you set up powerful conflicts. You have given yourself the freedom to overeat, but it's killing you!

The freedom of self-discipline is real freedom. It brings security, stability, self-understanding, and achievement. You can develop a positive craving for the freedom of self-discipline, and when you have it, there is no room in your life for other compulsions; you are safe. You can see that, can't you?

What have you done right today? You have seen that out-of-control eating is not freedom but the worst kind of slavery. You acknowledge that the freedom of self-discipline is the freedom you crave.

Today's Action Plan: I will be free of my food compulsion. I will fight through to a winner's self-control.

Beginnings

We may our ends by our beginnings know.
Sir John Denham

Make a good beginning because beginnings are tied to endings. The longest journey, as the Chinese proverb says, begins with the first step, so make that step a good one. Don't be wishy-washy about your commitment. Don't hedge. Don't say, "I'll try." Say, "I'll do it." Action is commitment, don't you agree?

Since you are a new person every day, you must renew your commitment every day. Each morning as you read from this book, or from the original *Thin Book*, commit yourself to living without excess food. Do that so that you can walk forward to the winner's circle.

If you had a slip yesterday, give yourself another chance today — give yourself a thousand times a thousand chances. The only failure is in punishing yourself for a stumble, self-destructively taking away a new chance for a positive life.

Remember that beginnings and endings are related. If you want a happy ending, make a happy beginning. Go joyously to work on yourself. There's so much to learn, so much to do — more than you can imagine. When your body and mind are not weighed down with too many calories, mountainous problems become little ant-hills. Make a good beginning today, won't you?

What have you done right today? You have given yourself a good beginning, which is the first step to a happy ending. You see that one good step at a time, one good day at a time, can change your life.

Today's Action Plan: I will recommit myself to a winner's life. I will make a good beginning.

April 23

Every Little Thing

The whole is greater than the sum of its parts.
General Systems Theory

If you didn't take physics, you missed an idea that could
be useful to you — the General Systems Theory. Overeaters are often impatient people; we want what we
want, and we want it *right now.* We'd just as soon skip
over all the little details of the Twelve Action MindSteps,
and get right to the good part, the part where we lose all
our weight and live healthy and happy (and wealthy
too) forever after. You've got every right to yearn for the
good life, but achievement is the result of putting all the
right parts together so that the whole emerges. You can
agree so far, can't you?

All the little parts of the winning puzzle that you read
about so far are necessary to the whole. None of the
MindSteps is the answer by itself, but all of them
together make the whole winning life possible. Read
them over at least once a day, especially if you're having
trouble. If you're mired in problems, chances are you've
forgotten the basics. Use the MindSteps not as a gospel
but as a checklist or a road map. Review them so you
can check your position to see that you're still on course.
You'll do that today, won't you?

What have you done right today? You have learned
the relationship of all the small parts of your plan to the
whole. Each one is important to complete the picture of
success, your success.

**Today's Action Plan: I will remember that all the parts
of my winning plan have to be in place before the whole
picture emerges. I will read the MindSteps.**

Who's Responsible for Your Weight?

It is in the ability to deceive oneself that the greatest talent is shown.

Anatole France

There are a hundred theories about how people become overweight in the first place. It doesn't matter which one eventually proves correct. Right now, today, you are responsible for your weight. You own it. You, only you, can deal with it — not your doctor, your family, your friends, or members of your support group. Will you be happy about that?

Let's see why you should love to be responsible for your own weight. If others are responsible, then someone or something is in control of your life. If you are responsible, then you are in control. You, no one and nothing but you, controls your life. Believe that. It takes the mystery out of weight loss and maintenance and puts you in charge of your own success.

This concept — that you have the power of control in your life — sounds simple. You think you understand, but this simplest of all ideas is the most difficult to grasp.

What does having control mean? It means that what you think and what you do control the way you feel. Have you got that? Does it keep slipping away from you? Try hard to accept it. Winners base their entire lives on this concept. You can too, can't you?

What have you done right today? You have owned yourself. You are ready to take the mystery out of achievement and put in your own control. That's freedom!

Today's Action Plan: I will own my weight. I will take the power to act into my own hands. I will accept help, but when it comes to doing — it's all up to me.

April 25

The Right Moves

Pick any time that suits your schedule and your needs. The important thing is to make it a regular routine. We are creatures of habit. So let the force of habit help you maintain your exercise program.

Dr. Kenneth H. Cooper

Are you making the right moves? Weight maintenance is based on the laws of thermodynamics — energy in equals energy out. So why not put more emphasis on the energy-out side of the equation? So many overweight people overlook physical movement as the most positive form of weight control. You'd like to be one of those who make the right moves, wouldn't you?

There's another aspect of exercise you may not have considered. Exercise changes your self-image from an immobile, sedentary person to an active, moving person. Visualize yourself running, jogging, swimming, bicycling.

You're exhilarated, and you look great! You like that picture, don't you?

The average person (thin or overweight) doesn't stick to exercise. Half who start a program drop out within a year. But you're not average. And you know vigorous exercise helps you lose weight even if you don't lower your food intake further. Every exercise works for somebody. Find the ones that work for you and stick to them. You gave up striving for average and decided to exercise like a winner. Say YES to exercise. Say YES to life. Do it today, won't you?

What have you done right today? You have looked at the energy equation and decided to be on the side of the winners. Congratulations!

Today's Action Plan: I will make the right moves. I will be one of the winners in life. Make room for me!

April 26

Anger = Lost Energy

Anger is a short madness.

Horace

Of all the emotional energy available to overeaters, anger is often the most ill-spent. In this world full of frustrations, anger is a normal reaction. For instance, if someone was deliberately cruel or falsely accused you, you had a right to be angry. But you'd rather handle that legitimate anger in constructive ways, wouldn't you?

First, be prepared for less than perfect treatment from others. It's not always a fair world, so if you don't expect too much fairness, you won't be outraged when someone is inconsiderate.

Second and more important, don't turn your anger on yourself. When things go wrong, they aren't always your fault. Turning your anger inward is a way to avoid confronting others. It *is* easier but the results are disastrous. Do you think you have no right to be angry because you're overweight? What nonsense!

If your anger is appropriate, then get it out and get it over. Face the source of your anger. Tell your oppressor, "I don't like that."

Everything negative that happens to you is not your fault because you are overweight. You do have a right to be angry. Remember that, won't you?

What have you done right today? You've learned to confront anger instead of letting it simmer. You realize that your weight has nothing to do with your rights to human feelings of frustration.

Today's Action Plan: I will not expect the world to treat me with kid gloves. I will not turn anger against myself.

Never Bored

I may be unhappy with myself, but at least I'm never bored while I'm eating.
Overheard at a diet group

You have three enemies that can destroy the best plan for right-eating, that can disrupt your schedule to lose pounds or maintain a natural weight: boredom, fatigue, and hunger. They are three villains lurking on every overeater's path to achievement. Let's look at them one at a time for the next three days to see what you can do to turn these small traps into big triumphs. You're ready for some new insights, aren't you?

Overeaters often eat to excess to fill time. Unfilled time allows too much opportunity for unpleasant emotions to surface. Thoughts of unmet responsibilities and a hundred guilts and fears can rise up to haunt you. But eating is no way to resolve negative feelings about yourself.

It's hard to be bored if you are following the Action life demanded by the achiever's schedule. You're just too busy. It takes time to come to self-understanding. It takes time to find the proper eating plan for reaching and maintaining your natural weight. It takes time to exercise for a lean, high-energy body. The achieving life is crammed to the brim with positive mental and physical activity. Winners are seldom bored. And you are a winner, aren't you? The correct answer is YES.

What have you done right today? You know that boredom is empty time filled with negative feelings and behavior, and signals a need for change. You know that Action is never boring.

Today's Action Plan: I will be too busy to be bored. Boredom is an excuse to overeat, and I will not use this excuse again.

Never Too Tired

But at the end of the day, I was too tired to prepare the proper foods.
Overheard at a diet group

Winners plan ahead. It really is that simple. You are serious about losing weight, so you give it top priority. You know the foods you need to eat. You make them easily available so you won't grab high-calorie snacks to get over the fatigue slump. You're doing all these things, aren't you?

Ignoring your need for the food on your plan does not de-emphasize food. Instead, it sabotages your program. When you're tired, the temptation to reach for the nearest food is far stronger than when you're rested.

Program some relaxation into every day. This prevents you from getting so tired that you resort to the old food pacifier. A complete weight-loss program includes relaxation as an important part of the day. If you are getting too tired to maintain smart eating habits, change your schedule. Remember when something doesn't work, change it. Winners do that. Be a winner.

Most of us overeaters convince ourselves that we save time by grabbing the first food at hand. Too often this means slipping into a binge. But the binge/guilt pattern never saves time, does it? You do admit the truth of that, don't you?

What have you done right today? You realize that fatigue leads to overeating. You see the importance of planning ahead and keeping the foods you need close at hand. You're acting more like a winner every day.

Today's Action Plan: I will not allow myself to get too tired. I will not use fatigue as an excuse to overeat.

Never Too Hungry

I skipped breakfast, and by lunch I was ready to eat everything in the house.

Diet club member

Many dieters think if they're not hungry, the diet isn't working. This is as silly as believing a medicine won't cure if it isn't bitter. If you have a nutritionally balanced eating plan, you should be hungry at meal times, but not too hungry. You have such an eating plan, don't you?

Don't skip meals. Nothing — absolutely nothing — is more important to your high-energy Action life than nourishing, tasty meals.

Listen to your body. It is always sending you messages if you will just listen. If you want to eat at six o'clock every evening, then do so — every evening. Don't try to set some arbitrary time for meals that doesn't correspond to your body's needs. If your family has to eat earlier or later, let them, at least until you can gradually wean your body from its preferred time.

The point is, for an overeater, getting too hungry is dangerous. Take whatever steps you must to avoid it. Will you do this for yourself? Say YES. Please.

What have you done right today? You are learning what you must do to achieve your goals. You have a winner's curiosity and determination. Good for you.

Today's Action Plan: I will not allow myself to get too hungry. I will plan meals so I won't have an excuse to overeat.

April 30

Where You Are and Where You're Going

milestone: an important event or turning point
Webster's Dictionary

One third of the year has passed. How has it gone for you?

Have you let it slip away, one day at a time, taking with it forgotten or broken promises that you made to yourself? Or have you fanned the flame — your own pilot-light of hope — into a fire that has warmed your life and lighted your way to achievement you never before thought possible for you? Which has it been?

Each day your dream is alive. It's just as strong today as it was on January 1. Each day you are new. And you are capable. Lack of capability never was and never will be your problem.

A life of overeating suffocates. It has results that have names: grief, confusion, anger, body-guilt.

A winning, achieving life has fantastic rewards that have names too: self-esteem, self-understanding, confidence, courage, authority.

The choice is yours. It's your choice today. It will be your choice every day of this year, every day of your life. Only you can truly put the MindSteps into Action. Don't drift aimlessly. Make Action your rudder to help you steer a straight course. Have you made that YES decision about your life? Say it — YES.

What have you done right today? If nothing else, you have read this page. You have kept the light of hope glowing. You realize you have the ability. Now put it into Action.

Today's Action Plan: I will fan the flame of hope. I hereby say YES to a winner's life.

A Debt You Don't Owe

Worry is interest paid on trouble before it falls due.
William Inge

Get ready. You've got work to do today: uncover a layer of self-deception, give up a negative illusion, expose a false fear. Don't stand still while your life marches by. Use your imprisoned energy to get into Action. Get ready, won't you?

We overeaters are often over-worriers, especially when our eating is out of control. We tend to "terrible-ize" the future because the present is so awful. Our negative fantasy destroys our chances for success. It's self-destructive. Do you ever "terrible-ize" what's yet to happen?

When you worry about imaginary trouble, you believe in false limits. Life self-limited by worry is closed to achievement.

Every day build positive expectations of the future. Always expect to win and you increase the odds in your favor. That's perfectly clear, isn't it?

What have you done right today? You have faced a tendency to worry. You are ready to discard the limitations you inflicted on yourself. Take charge today, and you won't be afraid of tomorrow.

Today's Action Plan: I will not "terrible-ize" the future. I will not limit my life with false fears.

The Big Sell-out!

One is never too old to yearn.
Italian Proverb

Have you denied your potential with an age excuse? Perhaps you said, "If I were younger, I could lose weight." Or, "If I were older, I could control my overeating." Have you ever used age as an excuse for not making a commitment to an achieving life?

Some people never seem to be the right age to do anything. Why should overweights slam the door to a thinner body with this flimsy excuse? Why miss an opportunity by putting age limits on achievement?

Age is no barrier to a winning life. You can get the Action habit at sixteen or sixty. Being a winner can mean wonderful, positive things: more admiration, self-esteem, respect; less fear, failure, and worries. Winning brings happiness and satisfaction to your life beyond anything you ever dreamed. You're not too old or too young for those benefits, are you?

Failure is fed by excuses; winning is fed by knowing and doing what's important to you. You know what's important to you today, don't you?

What have you done right today? You have seen that never being just the "right age" is a ticket to a self-limited life. You've decided to get the Action habit, whatever your age.

Today's Action Plan: I will not allow age to be a barrier to my winning life. I am the perfect age to win, right now!

The Advance Guard of Winning

The first principle of achievement is mental attitude.
Man begins to achieve when he begins to believe.
J. C. Roberts

You can't wish away extra pounds. But did you know you can believe them away? Say YES right here to this important idea. There's a simple explanation about why belief is perhaps the most powerful of all mental attitudes. Strong belief in a goal propels you into Action, and your belief communicates confidence to others. They feed this positive energy back to you, further increasing your belief in yourself — a marvelous merry-go-round. You see that so far, don't you?

Believe you will succeed. Believe you will lose weight, take charge of your life, and get on the winner's path. Look at the really successful people around you. What do you see? They have an I'm-going-to-be-the-best attitude, don't they? If you check further, chances are they aren't smarter than you, nor do they have any secret door open for them. Chances are, the difference is their powerful belief that they will succeed.

Begin to believe that nothing can keep you overweight. This one basic belief will power your mind. Your mind will then begin to attract and develop Action answers. Before you know it you'll be on a winning streak. What does it matter if you've tried before and failed? This time you will go beyond anything you've ever done. Believe it, won't you?

What have you done right today? You have learned that believing is the most positive power you can use. Like perpetual motion, your belief sends out waves of confidence which come back as others' belief in *you*. Keep believing!

Today's Action Plan: I believe I can lose weight. I know I can keep a healthy weight as long as I believe.

May 4

Yesterday's Ghosts

Until you learn to name your ghosts and to baptize your hopes, you have not yet been born; you are still the creation of others.

Marie Cardinal

Put names to your ghosts. Learn what your fears are, as the fourth Action MindStep says. When you do this, you can recognize your wants (hopes). Free from fear and armed with legitimate hopes, you can recreate yourself. You can be reborn in a new likeness, in a new body and mind that you will be proud of. You are ready to be born again, aren't you?

There is a place that only your unique self can fill. Think about it. Imagine yourself in that place. Believe you can reach it. Encourage yourself. Don't compete with others, compete with yourself. Actually the only person you have to best is your "yesterday" self. You can beat yesterday, can't you? Yes, it is that simple. Accept today's hopes and recognize the effort you put into today's improvement.

Above all, on this day, respect yourself. You are uniquely wonderful: no one else in this world can be like you. Because you try, each day you win a little more. Put names to yesterday's fears: call them indecision, bingeing, no-goals. They are only ghosts today. You have banished them with your commitment, haven't you?

What have you done right today? You encouraged yourself as only you can. You named your fears and they are gone.

Today's Action Plan: I will get rid of the fear ghosts. I will baptize my hope in commitment to goals.

Finding Assets in Negative Places

We shall not cease from exploration . . .
                                                    T. S. Eliot

You can find assets in unexpected places which will help you reach your goals. Most overeaters are extremely self-critical. Are you one of these? The next time you start berating yourself, look at your supposed liabilities with a positive eye. You'll do this, won't you?

Let's say you are a fussy housekeeper or office worker. That's a negative, isn't it? Not necessarily. The positive side is that you are very exact. Possibly, when you haven't a goal to work toward, you are fussy for the sake of fussiness. When you have a goal — a goal of thinness — your behavior changes from fussiness to exactness.

If you tend to become negatively over-involved, a goal will transform that liability into the asset of focused energy. If you have been an angry person, a goal will transform that liability into the asset of assertiveness. Do you see the possibilities when you look at yourself positively?

Turn your liabilities into assets, your problems into challenges. Say YES, won't you?

What have you done right today? By adding a goal, you have taken character problems and turned them into assets and challenges. You have seen that goals can turn a self-defeating course into a path to the winner's circle.

Today's Action Plan: I will turn my liabilities into assets. I will look at the positive side of my behavior.

Action Means You Have Been Energized

*We act ourselves into ways of believing and believe
ourselves into ways of acting.*
Joseph Chilton

Thinking is preparation for Action. But Action must follow thought, or the thought is wasted. "I'll think about this weight goal," you say. But thinking isn't Action. "All right, I'll try," you venture, going a step further. Trying is not Action either. Sorry, no failure-insurance: "Well, I tried, didn't I?" Just thinking or trying isn't enough, is it?

Think, decide, then act. Take specific Action. Create opportunities for success whether your goal is ten pounds or one hundred pounds.

Yes, there's a risk of failure with commitment. Take that risk. Failing only means you have more to learn; it doesn't mean you're finished. If you've stumbled, you've learned something. Don't ever proclaim inadequacy or predict failure by saying, "I'm no good. I always fail."

Predict success. You must keep believing, no matter what, and you will reach your weight goal. Nothing can stop you. Make that commitment now, won't you?

What have you done right today? You have seen that thinking and trying are not Action. Commitment together with Action is the only way to get on the path to your goal. Of course you can do it.

Today's Action Plan: I will take Action on my weight goal. I will risk anything but the risk of not beginning.

The Sugar Monster

The more sugar you eat in a lifetime, the more
abnormal your response to sugar becomes.

Dr. Robert Atkins

Are you addicted to refined sugar? Does one bite of a
sweet mean that you'll probably eat to the bottom of the
container?

Can you eat half a candy bar, fold the paper over it,
and put it away? Do you use sugar as emotional
therapy, running to it as to a lover, friend, or comforter
whenever you're under stress? After eating a lot of
refined sugar, do you have headaches, drowsiness, bloat-
ing, weeping spells, a hung-over feeling the next day?
Are you saying, "Yes!"?

It's terribly important that you answer these questions
about you and sugar with candor. Are you ready to face
the sugar monster honestly? Listen to your body. What
is it telling you about your use of refined sugar?

If you were just an average sweet-user and could cut
out refined sugar for one year, you would rid your body
of the caloric equivalent of fifty pounds. Think about it.
Please! If you are a true addict, getting rid of sugar
completely is the only way to bring your addiction under
control.

You are restating your resolve every day, aren't you?
Today, when you declare your burning desire to be thin
and healthy, you and you alone can make a crucial YES
decision to get the sugar monster off your back. Take
Action, won't you?

What have you done right today? You faced the fact
that refined sugar is a barrier to the kind of achieving life
you want. Yes, it was tough, but you faced it squarely.

**Today's Action Plan: I will evaluate honestly what my
body is telling me about refined sugar. If I am addicted, I
will cease to be a sugar-junkie.**

What Do You Want?

What you should want more than the habit is the benefit of giving it up.

José Silva

What do you want more than anything in the world? Say it out loud. Did you wish for something like this: to lose weight and maintain my weight goal; to become a dynamic, achieving winner for the rest of my life. Is that about what you said?

Your wish will be granted if you follow seven basic, powerful ideas. Don't be fooled by their simplicity; they will take all your strength to achieve — not more strength than you have, but all that you have. They are:

1. Define what you want.
2. Live intensely with that idea.
3. Become thin in your own mind first.
4. Visualize yourself at your natural weight.
5. Don't carry around negative emotional baggage.
6. Practice consistent positive affirmation of yourself.
7. Put it all into Action.

Do you recognize the power in those ideas? If you do what it takes to become who you want to become, you *will* become that person. Although the words are different, some of these ideas appear in the most ancient philosophies. They may not be the newest, but they are probably the most avoided, most unused great ideas in the world. Today, they're all yours to use, aren't they?

What have you done right today? You discovered a way to state what you want, powerful ideas which can open the world of achievement to you.

Today's Action Plan: I will define what I want to be. Then I will win, using the the oldest ideas in the world.

How to Build Up a Good Head of Self-esteem

*Self-reverence, self-knowledge, self-control. These three
alone lead life to sovereign power.*
Alfred, Lord Tennyson

Pop psychology aside, nobody else can hand you self-esteem; not a parent, not a mate, not a friend. Only *you*
can give yourself the gift of self-esteem because only
your opinion counts when it comes to self-esteem. If you
don't like yourself, well, it doesn't seem to matter who
else does or doesn't. So like yourself. That's all there is
to self-esteem. That's all. Liking yourself. Simple, isn't it?

Now comes the question: how do you go about liking
yourself? This, too, is not complex. You like yourself
when you do what you know you should do, which
makes you feel good about yourself. You make YES
decisions, not NO decisions. You begin to feel even
better. Self-esteem means you are happily involved with
yourself — not morbidly or obsessively, as in the past,
but happily as you are right now.

For centuries self-love was discouraged, but you've
learned that lesson far too well. Because you have a
problem with overweight, you may need to change your
pattern of thinking about yourself. Whisper it, so that
someday you may shout it. Say, "I like myself!" There,
that felt good, didn't it?

What have you done right today? You have discov-ered that liking yourself is inextricably linked with how
effective you are. And how effective you are determines
how well you will lose weight and keep it off.

Today's Action Plan: I will build up a good head of
self-esteem, liking myself more today than I did yester-day. I will forge strong links between liking myself and
my eating plan so that one day I will know what it is to
love myself.

If You Love Discipline — Smile

Without discipline, one can only stare like a window-shopper at the good things in life, and shrug, and move on . . .

Amy Gross

A photographer has a trick for getting his stone-faced subjects to smile for the camera. "If you love sex," he shouts, "smile!" Invariably a grin spreads across the subject's face. What if the photographer had said: "If you love discipline, smile!" Those portraits would be grim, wouldn't they? Now, if you stepped into the picture, you'd have an automatic, huge grin for discipline, wouldn't you?

When you stopped overeating and began to achieve the winning, thinning life, you realized that daily discipline was absolutely necessary to your happiness. One of the major ingredients of your success became a structured life.

Without discipline, you flail about, wasting time, picking up this and dropping that. You've learned that, haven't you? You found there is nothing more comforting and comfortable than a day based on doing what you know you should do, when you know you should do it. Such a day is enough to make you smile, isn't it?

What have you done right today? You have reinforced your own daily discipline; you put structure into your day to make it better. You have seen that the way to achieve what you want is to go after it systematically. No wonder you're smiling!

Today's Action Plan: I will be a disciplined doer, not a window-shopper in life. I will love a structured day.

Disguised

*. . . without my magic cloak of blubber and invisibility,
I felt naked, pruned as though some essential covering
was missing.*
                                                    Margaret Atwood

One of the awful mysteries of overweight is to lose
excess weight — even hundreds of pounds — only to
regain it all with, perhaps, a ten-pound bonus. This is
the infamous yo-yo syndrome, with the yo-yo bouncing
back ever higher. Nothing is more painful than the
hopelessness and shame of regaining all your lost weight.
Can you think of anything worse?

Yet, surprisingly, some people who have gone through
this tragedy talk about not feeling comfortable with their
thin bodies, of looking in the mirror and not recognizing
themselves. Unfortunately the longer you've been overweight, the harder it is to get rid of the fat self-image —
even when you are at a weight natural for you. When
your internal image isn't reflected in your mirror, you
have a distorted self-image.

One way to prevent the yo-yo syndrome is to convince yourself that you deserve to be thin. Now is the
time to discard your overweight self-image and develop a
solid understanding of your unique worth. And it is
possible when you approach your new LifeWay with
intensity — a combination of attention and concentration. You've been doing that every day for months now,
haven't you?

What have you done right today? You have discovered that you cannot disguise yourself from yourself.
You see the necessity of adjusting your inner image, so it
will be comfortable with the new thin body you will
have. And you'll have it soon.

**Today's Action Plan: I will not hide inside my excess
pounds. My inner mirror will reflect my true image.**

Get a Mentor

If you want success, copy from someone.
W. Clement Stone

People in the business world offer mutual support by networking; working with a group of supportive people who can help you make good career decisions. Often there is one special person, someone older perhaps, or more experienced, or someone with the kind of success you want: a mentor. One who will guide you by showing you the best way to achieve. Successful diet groups have mentors. In Overeaters Anonymous they're called sponsors. They give encouragement, direction, and strength to fellow overeaters. A mentor sounds like a good idea, doesn't it?

Choose a good mentor (or more than one) and then imitate their success, adapt their methods to your needs. The important thing is that you'll be imitating success.

Successful people are easy to recognize. They're the ones who don't talk a good job, they do a good job; they don't just think about losing weight, they lose weight. These are people you can honestly admire because they've turned their lives around. Success shines so brightly, you can't miss it.

People tend to band together. They like to be with other people. Go ahead, find your group; go immediately to where the winners are. That makes sense to you, doesn't it?

What have you done right today? You have decided to imitate success, to seek out the doers in life and to imitate them.

Today's Action Plan: I will find a mentor. I will listen to what he or she tells me, and do it.

One Day at a Time

The future belongs to those who live intensely
in the present.

Anonymous

The Anonymous groups (Alcoholics Anonymous is the oldest), which offer hope and recovery to alcoholics and other drug-dependents, overeaters, and gamblers, teach that no one can live any time except now. Yesterday is a cancelled check, tomorrow is a promissory note, but today is cash that you can spend. You agree with this philosophy, don't you?

It's important to you that you do agree. Far too many compulsive people try to live in every time but right now. They drag yesterday around, moaning about what they did wrong. They worry about repeating yesterday's mistakes tomorrow. Today is totally lost while they fret about the past and fear the future. Life just passes them by, a day at a time.

Today is the only day you can do anything about. Use it. Make it work for you. By the time you go to bed tonight, be one day closer to achieving a thinner body, self-understanding, and a high-energy, enthusiastic life. Create a chance for yourself today by concentrating all your desire into the next few hours. Do it, won't you?

What have you done today? You have released yesterday and tomorrow and focused on today. You have learned that you can use each day only once.

Today's Action Plan: I will take life one day at a time. At the end of the day, I will be closer to my goal.

Affirm Yourself

Believe you can, or believe you can't; either way you'll be right.

Henry Ford

You can respond two ways to a compliment: with self-affirmation or self-criticism. When a friend says, "You were great!" you can say, "Thank you, I'm pleased with my job too" or "Oh, that's nothing." Which do you want: an active inner criticizer or a healthy inner affirmer?

Don't brush aside compliments as if they were untrue, of no consequence. Accept the validation of others. Believe that you are worthy.

Your criticizer also erodes your self-esteem when you tell yourself, "You're so stupid!" Be more self-encouraging. Tell yourself, "I am fun to be around" or "I really did a great job that time." It's important to affirm your own strength, to give yourself compliments you richly deserve. Now honestly, haven't you been more generous with strangers than with yourself?

What have you done right today? You learned to listen to your self-affirmer. Today you affirmed that: "I'm really doing a good job putting all the MindSteps into Action. I'm fun to be with today."

Today's Action Plan: I will overwhelm my criticizer with self-affirmation. I will compliment myself at least once today.

The Success of Failure

We are all failures — at least the best of us are.
James M. Barrie

No matter how hard people try, failures happen, and overeaters have their share. How many times have you said, "Oh, I'm no good. I've failed again"? You'd like a way to take the fail out of failure, wouldn't you?

Don't view failure as a catastrophe that happens only to you. Failure is part of playing to win. If you get in the game, you might drop the ball.

Never see a failure as losing the whole ball game. View it as simply gaining information you need to change your methods. Failure is just a new set of instructions to help you reach your goal.

Never let one failure make you quit reaching for success. Value the chance you have been given to perfect your understanding of the Twelve Action MindSteps. Take it as an opportunity to practice your positive mental techniques and perfect your performance for the next confrontation. Think of what you've learned, not what you've lost. That's the difference between winning and failing, isn't it?

What have you done right today? You learned how to squeeze success out of failure. You learn what you can from failure, so that next time you'll be wiser and tougher. There is absolutely no way you can fail with this way of thinking.

Today's Action Plan: I will take the fail out of failure. I will focus on the positive future, not the negative past.

Yes, You Can Do More

Do more than exist, live.
                                    John H. Rhoades

Are you doing all you can to get a thin winner's body? No matter what your answer, you can do more. Yes, you can. There is no limit to how much you can improve. When you ask how to find ways to increase achievement, you open your mind to answers. Try it. You haven't reached the limit of your capacity. Your capacity to achieve expands every day when you follow your energizing new LifeWay. Successful people have a simple formula for daily achievement: Do what you do well even better, and try to do even more of it every day. You could do just a *little* more, couldn't you?

Do more than be aware of your feelings about over-eating; understand them. Do more than be mildly curious; look around you. Do more than read about nutrition; make this knowledge a part of you. Do more than hear; listen for meaning. Do more than think; put your thoughts into Action. You can do a little more of everything that you do because you are capable, aren't you? Say YES.

You can do all these things. What you want you can achieve. What you desire, you deserve. You are worth far more to the world than you realize. Increasingly your life will be better if that's what you want. Do more, won't you?

What have you done right today? You learned that achievers don't put limits on success; they believe they can do a little more each day. You are an achiever. You can do a little more each day and build a whole new life.

Today's Action Plan: I will do what I do well even better. I will do a little more of it today.

From the Neck up

*Fat people often think of themselves solely in terms of
the "neck up." Their bodies are disowned, alienated,
foreign, perhaps stubbornly present but not truly a part
of the real self.*

Marcia Millman

Do you resist buying clothes for yourself until you look
just right? Do you wear the same threadbare clothes
because you can't face the thought of shopping for new
clothes for your hated body? If you answered yes, you
are cooperating with your inner critic's campaign to
bring you down. This is possible, isn't it?

You are important. Important enough to look your
best every day, no matter what your present weight. To
feel important, look important, and dress as if today will
be the most successful day of your life.

You need to look important to others, so they will
mirror that back to you. But even more, you need to
look important for yourself. A good appearance talks to
you. It helps you to think on a higher level, to risk
more, change more.

When you look in the mirror, your image should say,
"You are important, intelligent and achieving. You lead a
high-energy life, and by the way, haven't you lost weight
lately?" Say YES to that.

What have you done right today? You have dressed to
reflect how important you are. It's about time.

**Today's Action Plan: I will honor myself by dressing
well today. My appearance will say to me that I am an
important person.**

Now Is the Time

One of these days is none of these days.
H. G. Bohn

Today is the day. This minute is the time. It seems that one deadly phrase pays the rent for half the world's psychiatrists, "If only . . . ." People who constantly mutter, "If only . . . ," have never learned to give themselves a next time. They are stuck in regret, unable to see the opportunities around them. You aren't an "If only . . . " person, are you?

You've got work to do today. You have a goal to pursue, a plan to put into Action, an idea to work on, a problem to solve, a decision to make. You are too busy *doing* to be an "If only . . . " person.

Using the present is the admission ticket to a full life. Use your *now.* Don't procrastinate your life away. Get rid of your favorite excuses for postponing living — lack of money, support, talent, tools. You have all you need — the desire to achieve a whole life, to be a thinner winner.

Resolve to use every hour, every minute of this day. "One of these days" is here now, isn't it?

What have you done right today? You have recognized "If only . . . " as the cry of dreams never launched, goals never pursued, projects never started. You will not poison your life with "If only . . . ."

Today's Action Plan: I will not postpone a minute of my life. I will take Action now to get where I want to go.

A Two-minute Picture of You

He who values himself is valued.

Anonymous

Here's a written guarantee: Practice the Twelve Action MindSteps and you will gain a new best friend, yourself. We overeaters get so low in self-esteem that it's difficult to do good things for ourselves. Value yourself. Today, even though you haven't quite accepted the idea yet, treat yourself like a new person, won't you?

- Act as if you value, not hate, yourself; as if you understand, not despise, yourself.
- Act as if you are poised, not tense; confident, not confused; bold, not timid.
- Act as if you are full of enthusiasm, not bored; achieving, not failing; energized, not tired.
- Act as if you are a positive person and you will become as you act.

The game of "act as if" works. You don't even have to believe at first; doing will create belief. Make your advantages a gift to you today: you are alive, you possess this minute, you are absolutely unique, and you are capable of more than you ever thought. So stop being your own victim and take charge of your dreams right now. They will come true when you really become your own best friend. Believe that, won't you?

What have you done right today? You are acting as if you already have everything you need to become a thinner winner. You do!

Today's Action Plan: I will value myself. I will act out and believe in this positive picture of myself.

Your Dream Come True

*The best way to make your dreams come true is to
wake up.*

George Alban

What is your biggest dream? What is the one thing in
this world you want most to attain? If you want to reach
and maintain your natural weight, you can see your
dream come true. One of the basic principles of Action
(incorporated in the twelfth MindStep) is always play to
win. Only when your creative energies are propelled by
a winning dream can you get going and keep going. You
agree with that so far, don't you?

Do you care about your body enough? Do you
believe that you deserve the body you want? You must
love yourself enough to give yourself your dream. Then
you must put it into Action. Be wide-awake to every
opportunity. You choose how to lead your life, but if
you play life to win, your dreams come true.

Winning begins with hope, but you must supply the
Action to motivate it. What is your hope? That you will
be free of the terrible nightmare of overeating, and wake
up to a happy, winning life? Soon this hope will come
true, won't it? Say YES.

What have you done right today? You learned to be
awake to your dreams, to use them to fuel Action. You
want to lose your excess weight and play life to win.

**Today's Action Plan: I will put my dreams into
Action. I will win my fondest dream.**

What Does Success Mean?

There is no upper limit to what individuals are capable of doing with their minds. There is no age limit that bars them from beginning. There is no obstacle that cannot be overcome if they persist and believe.

E. F. Wells

This is a book of happy changes that lead to success. How do you define success? Success is usually defined as the attainment of personal goals. You're not limited to just a weight goal — in fact such a limitation would probably be harmful to your reaching that goal. Most overeaters need to make big changes in attitude, outlook, and the way they respond to life. This is not a book of diet tricks, eating on small plates, keeping celery sticks ready at the front of the refrigerator. Those helpful ideas are covered elsewhere. The message in these pages is geared to do something else, to help you uncover the powerful person you didn't know existed, the person within you. You'd like to find that strong and happy person, wouldn't you?

You are making an investment in the present which will change your future. You are building an Action program of exercise, attitude, and right-eating for weight loss.

Today, you will travel as far as your inner ability will take you, and that is a great distance. You have no upper limit. You believe that, don't you?

What have you done right today? You see that your definition of success can expand as far as your commitment — endlessly.

Today's Action Plan: I will define what success means to me. I will open myself to change.

All or Nothing

*It's a common mistake to think of failure as the enemy
of success. Failure is a teacher — a harsh one,
but the best.*

Thomas J. Watson, Jr.

Do you know any all-or-nothing people? One little
mistake can lead them to abandon an entire project. If
you are such a person, one little bite can lead to an
overeating binge. Do you tend to see every bump in the
road as a good reason for taking a detour? All-or-
nothingism is a defeating mindset. You'd like to get rid
of it, wouldn't you?

If you take a bite of a food you've decided to
eliminate, usually something sweet, it's no reason to go
all the way; it's a reason to look for the reason. Analyze
that failure and make it work for you. Knowing why
you made an eating misstep will arm you if the same
problem arises again. Isn't this better than trying to blot
out the memory of a mistake with more calories?

All-or-nothingism is another form of perfectionism,
and perfectionism can undermine you. Determination to
be absolutely perfect can cause you to avoid any chance
of failure by setting no goals.

Small mistakes don't ruin your life any more than a
single bite ruins your fine eating plan. Think of mistakes
as a form of quick education and learn from them. If
you really profit from your mistakes, you'll reach your
life's goals faster. That's right, isn't it?

What have you done right today? You decided to let
go of the all-or-nothing habit. You're a quick learner!

**Today's Action Plan: I will profit from my mistakes. I
will learn from every misstep.**

Why Do You Binge?

*It was my worst binge, and I did it to myself. First I
made a mental list of all the "goodies" I'd been sacrificing
on my diet. Then I proceeded to eat my way
through the whole list.*
Joan P. at Overeaters Anonymous

We overeaters may begin a binge because we crave
certain foods, but we continue to binge because we don't
like ourselves enough to stop. Is that true for you?

Joan's basic problem was attitude: she didn't rejoice
about being rid of undesirable sweet foods, she thought
of her abstinence as a "sacrifice." Sacrifice is a powerful
negative word for overeaters. Sacrifices are for martyrs,
not overeaters.

Like many overweights, Joan was defiant, resistant,
angry, and frustrated — not a frame of mind conducive
to achievement. Joan didn't expect much success, and she
didn't have any.

Make a mental list of the new goals you want to
attain. Expect to get them! People usually get what they
expect. Joan prepared for a binge, she got one, and along
with her three-day binge a thirteen-pound weight gain.

Make positive, goal-directed lists. Expect the best from
yourself. You will, won't you?

What have you done right today? You have learned a
fascinating truth, you get what you expect. You learned
that binges are usually attitude problems, dangerously
coupled with self-hate. Expect no more binges!

Today's Action Plan: Of my own free will, I will get
rid of all mental binge lists. I will make constructive,
goal-directed lists.

Chain-eating

I was never too full. Even after I ate until I was sick, I still had an empty, gnawing feeling in the pit of my stomach.
A woman at Overeaters Anonymous

Are you a chain-eater? Do you respond to everything in life, from tragedy to ecstatic happiness, from fear to boredom, by overeating? Like the chain-smoker who lights a cigarette from the butt of one just smoked, a chain-eater reaches for a second snack while swallowing the first one. A few overeaters chain-eat all day, almost every day, while others chain-eat occasionally during highly emotional periods, but all overeaters are chain-eaters at some time. Why? You'd like to know why, wouldn't you?

Chain-eaters are not at peace with their bodies. They interpret every body-signal as a demand for food, then feel trapped by an insatiable appetite. Every discomfort, every emotion, every empty minute is translated into a physical need for food.

Get to know all your body's moods. Your body doesn't only hunger, it also wants activity, change, and rest. Nourish all your body's real wants. Feed them with your Action program.

The time-of-your-life is too important to smother with overeating. You see that clearly. Your destiny is in your control. Whatever will be is whatever you will it to be. That's first-class thinking, isn't it?

What have you done right today? You examined chain-eating and decided it is a destructive response to emotions and misread body-signals. You concluded that you must respond only to your body's real hunger to achieve an energized, winning life. Right again!

Today's Action Plan: I will translate boredom and anxiety as a need to get into Action. I will "feed" my positive wants.

The Three *Mess*-keteers

Things like sugar, salt, and fats simply weren't available to us in any quantity during the period of our genetic development. We can't handle them in more than trace quantities without causing a malfunction in our basic metabolic systems.

Robert Rodale

Sweets, salty snacks, and saturated fats are three "civilized foods" which can be harmful. Large quantities of this troublesome troika can make a mess of our metabolic systems. Most overweights (and thin people too) don't remember how pure food tastes. Junk food has spoiled our taste buds, hasn't it?

Sugar is Food Enemy Number One. Sucrose (sugar) becomes glucose in our bodies, overloads our pancreas, and in time causes a kind of endocrine burnout. Are you a sugarholic?

Salt is Food Enemy Number Two. It's implicated in the high blood pressure so many overweights suffer from. Most foods are over-salted in processing, cooking, and at the table. Are you a saltoholic?

Fat is Food Enemy Number Three. You may think you don't have a problem with fats. "I didn't know," said one overeater, "until I had to go on a gall bladder diet, just how addicted to fats I was." Are you a fatoholic?

Make a decision to eliminate or cut down all three food enemies. Reclaim your taste buds. Retrain them to enjoy more subtle flavors. You're making good choices these days, aren't you?

What have you done right today? You have chosen to enjoy the natural flavors of food from now on. Good!

Today's Action Plan: I will eat for maximum health. I will explore alternatives to sugary, salty, fatty foods.

Always Go First Class

*You are what you think, you become what you think,
and what you think becomes reality.*

Anonymous

When you think about your life, always be a first-class thinker. Dream great dreams. The more success you want, the greater you'll have to think. Today and tomorrow are important, not yesterday. Forget yesterday and shed the anger you felt about how limited your life was. Focus on where you're going, not where you've been, won't you?

From now on, life is opportunity. Nothing is closed to you any more. The only limits are the ones in your own mind. Stretch your mind. Don't be afraid to shoot for the supposedly unattainable. Your true desire is within your grasp. Go straight to first-class goals. No second-class thinking for you!

Use a first-class vocabulary, words that promise achievement. Use words that create winning images: victory, happiness, hope, energy, Action. You've got the idea, haven't you?

What have you done right today? You bought a first-class ticket to the rest of your life. You decided that you can stretch the limits of your thinking to include anything you want.

Today's Action Plan: I will not sell myself short. I will imagine the greatest opportunity; then I will make it my goal.

You're Greater than You Think

To believe is to be strong. Doubt cramps energy.
Belief is power.

Frederick W. Robertson

It's hard to think of yourself as unique and wonderful if
your imagination is cramped by self-deprecation. It's a
shame how some overweights concentrate on self-criticism. Their attitudes are so negative they can't accept
one kind word for themselves, from themselves or
others. That's a crime, isn't it?

If you have trouble thinking kindly about yourself,
maybe your arithmetic is backwards. Practice addition,
and quit subtracting. Instead of devaluing your every
act, add value. This will fit your thinking to what you
truly are. If you can't believe in your uniqueness, act as
if you can. You can't act that way for very long without
beginning to like yourself better. Concentrate on your
assets as you become more accepting.

Ask yourself, "What can I do to make myself more
valuable today?" Tell yourself, "I am getting stronger. By
reading these pages aloud, I am adding constructive
thoughts to my mind. I am far better than I think I am."

Try it and see. You can win a new image of yourself,
a new peace within yourself, a new idea of what life can
be. Stretch your mind until you can see your unique
worth, won't you? Say YES. Louder, please.

What have you done right today? You learned that,
no matter where you are, you are now heading in the
right direction. You will no longer hold yourself back
from your own potential by devaluing yourself.

**Today's Action Plan: I will add value to what I do
today. I will concentrate on my assets.**

May 28

No Retreat

If you get into the habit of retreating from challenges,
you're just a sitting duck for regrets.
                                        Gail Godwin

All of life challenges you. But how did you meet the
challenges? Think back right now. What do you regret
most? Probably the challenges you did not meet, the
times you said, "I could never do that!" Are unmet
challenges what you most regret?

You said, "I could never do that!" because you
believed it was true. And it *was* true, because to meet
challenges, even the small ones of everyday life, you
need to believe in your own importance.

What a difference the last five months have made.
Every day, with these pages you have told yourself that
you're a first-class person, capable of far more than you
ever imagined. You've done a good job of selling
yourself on yourself.

Whatever your challenge today, believe that you can
do it. When you believe something can be done, your
mind and spirit find ingenious ways to accomplish the
job. Believing that you already have the solution opens
the door to solutions you didn't realize you had.

You're a can-do, it-will-work, let's-get-going kind of
person. What a difference these words make, don't they?

What have you done right today? You accepted every
challenge believing you could do the job. You recognized
that having a sense of your own worth opens the door to
solutions. Keep going!

Today's Action Plan: I won't retreat from any chal-
lenge. I will look for can-do solutions.

Cynicism Never Lost a Pound

Everything in the world is done by hope.
Martin Luther

Do you have the will to hope or are you caught in a bog of negative, cynical tradition? "I've tried them all," you say. "Diet, exercise, fad, trend — none of them work for me." You are overwhelming hope with negatives, and without hope there is only the morass of cynicism. Is that where you stand right now? Are you afraid to really give the Twelve Action MindSteps a chance?

If you're lost in destructive, despairing feelings, there is a way to get your hope back. Paraphrase Blaise Pascal's wager about the existence of God. Say, "I've got everything to win if the MindSteps work, and nothing to lose if they don't. So why not go along?"

Think of it. If you are truly emptied of hope, you have nowhere to go; a hopeless life can't get any worse. But you can trick the devils of doom and gloom by acting as if you had hope, and through acting, find it. This actually *is* a triumph for hope.

Hope is positive food for the mind. What your mind consumes today determines habits, attitudes, and capacity to change. The question isn't whether you'll change today. You will. The question is *how* you will change. Cynicism says the change will be destructive. Hope says the change will be constructive. You'll go along with hope, won't you?

What have you done right today? You know that you can win by feeding your mind hope. You're determined from now on to bet on yourself. And it's a sure thing that you're going to win that bet.

Today's Action Plan: I will drop a loser's cynicism. I will feed my mind the positive food of hope.

Get Ready, Get Set, Get Motivated

> *If it weren't for the group support, I don't think
> I could make it.*
>   Overeaters Anonymous Member

Rugged individualists, hermits, and lighthouse keepers
don't need the support of a group. But how many of
them are overweight? Support is essential to keep most
overeaters going once they're on the road back to
winning health. That support can come from one partner
or a whole group, as long as you have similar goals and
the necessary understanding of a shared experience.
Strange as it seems, no one can help an overeater like
another overeater. You can see that, can't you?

Humans are essentially tribal. Most of us enjoy company, but those in trouble really *need* company. If you
talk about a particular problem you're having, it helps a
great deal when someone in the group simply says, "I
know how you feel." Groups perform a valuable function for overeaters. Getting the motivation to begin a
weight-loss or exercise program can be easier than
keeping your motivation high. Groups help you stay
highly motivated.

It helps you to stay motivated if others are counting
on you, even if it's to open the meeting room or make
the coffee. Try several groups until you find the right
one for you. You'll know it when you find it, won't
you? Say YES.

What have you done right today? Whether you need a
whole group, or just another person to confide in, you
have decided to go out and get what you need.

**Today's Action Plan: I will look for people-support
for my program. I will find a group where, when I share
my experience, someone says, "Me, too."**

May 31

The Three-week Time Capsule

. . . it takes the body twenty-one days to accept
new behavior.

Dr. Susan Jones

Familiar scene: Your school reunion, birthday party,
important wedding, or some other big event is only two
weeks away. You climb on the bathroom scale to see
how much weight you have to lose to get into your
favorite dress. As the pound indicator swings past the
point you thought it would stop at, you panic. Next you
set an unrealistic goal, allow yourself too little time,
become discouraged, and binge. Then you either stay at
home on the big day or wear the same outfit as last year,
one you vowed you would never wear again. Does this
scene strike a memory chord?

Setting goals is what this book is all about, especially
Action MindStep the Ninth. Take weight loss, exercise,
and attitude changes in steps. Set small, realistic goals on
your way to the big goal.

Give every change in your life at least three weeks.
This is the time your body and mind need to adjust to
any change in behavior. If you get rid of sugar, your
body usually requires twenty-one days to accept the
change as natural.

Whether it's food or a character change, getting rid of
it for at least three weeks will more than likely break
your dependence on it. Try it and see, won't you?

What have you done right today? You've learned a
formula that will lead you to a leaner, more attractive
body — allowing sufficient time and setting reachable
goals. You decided to give each goal at least three weeks.

**Today's Action Plan: I will set a goal and allow three
weeks for change. Just for today, I will give myself the
time I need.**

Your Body

*A body is forsaken when it becomes a source of pain
and humiliation instead of pleasure and pride.*
Alexander Lowen

Your greatest task today is to create the best possible
environment to promote weight loss. Do you agree? All
right then, there is one path to take. The toughest, most
essential move for overeaters is to move away from a
pervasive sense of body-hate. But before you begin this,
you must be convinced that it is possible to change a bad
relationship with your body. You would really like to do
this, wouldn't you?

Your body's appearance is the result of a lifetime of
choices. When you change your choices, you change
your body. Of course, making changes is sometimes
painful, but change is your choice. There are two kinds
of pain, the hopeless pain of staying an overeater, or the
joyful pain of changing the what, how, and why you
eat.

Make the right eating choices beginning today and the
negative way you feel about your body will begin to
disappear. Isn't this what you really want, to feel
comfortable within your body?

Arm yourself with facts about nutrition and exercise,
whatever you need to know to make better choices for
your body today. Act on these facts. You're beginning to
do this right now, aren't you?

What have you done right today? You have ended a
painful estrangement from your body. From now on,
your body will reflect your good food and exercise
choices.

**Today's Action Plan: I will make a commitment to
befriend my body. My first act of friendship will be to
make the right choices for me.**

Hitting the Right Note

Many of us die with our music unplayed.
Mary Kay Ash

Two conflicting voices carry on constant tune-playing in your head. One chants, "Help me!" The other sings, "Don't be a crybaby!" Because these voices don't harmonize, we tend to ignore both when we should heed both. Will you do it ?

It takes courage to ask sincerely for help from your family, a supportive friend, doctor, or diet group. It takes courage, too, to stand firm and battle your food problem. You can see how either tune could be right, depending on where you are on the road to recovering from overeating, can't you?

Find the hero in yourself. This hero may reach out to others with an eating problem, to take and to give help. Or this hero may say, "I will summon the strength and knowledge within me to make my stand." Either way, your decision has made certain your theme song is played without interrupting static or sour notes.

Prepare for success. It's coming. When you do what you know you should do, success elects you to the winner's circle. Do you believe this? Say YES. You attract what you believe. You believe you are a hero, so you will act like a hero, won't you?

What have you done right today? You recognized each of the two voices searching for the hero in you. You have decided that when you listen to life's music, it will be *your* song.

Today's Action Plan: I will find the hero in myself. I will have the courage to either seek help or take an individual stand. I will do whatever I must to win a thinner body.

The Worst Excuse

An excuse is worse and more terrible than a lie;
for an excuse is a lie guarded.
Alexander Pope

"Both my parents are overweight." "There's been a recent death in my family." "I have too many money worries to handle all this." "Nobody likes me." For heaven's sake, who could blame such people for overeating? Certainly they have reasons to overeat. So convincing. So righteous. Such good excuses, right? Wrong!

A good excuse is the worst excuse of all, even though it has a core of truth. It is a powerful enemy of weight-goal achievement. You may really come from a fat family, you may have suffered a terrible pain lately, you may be seriously short of funds, or your social life may be depressing. But the more often you repeat your excuse, the more convinced you are that it is completely true. Such an excuse will defeat your efforts to lose weight. There it is — the "reason" for your overeating.

Throw away the notion that if only this problem — whatever it is — would disappear, you would be able to control your overeating. Negative nonsense! You're only making your problems worse when you put off taking charge of your eating.

Be fully alive. Get rid of your so-called good excuse today and take charge, won't you? YES is your only answer.

What have you done right today? You have seen that all excuses, good and bad, are damaging. You've made a YES decision to get rid of all excuses to overeat.

Today's Action Plan: I will get rid of all my excuses. I will be fully alive, fully in charge.

Anger

Anger is only one letter short of danger.

Anonymous

The overeater's personality has been defined as angry.
No wonder. Look at the way we overeaters are treated:
labeled, libeled, and laughed at! All true. But anger, even
righteous anger, is dangerous to an overeater. We don't
get even when we eat, only fat. We must learn to handle
anger in positive ways, wouldn't you say?

Successful people encounter embarrassing, depressing
situations. How do they handle them? Confident, achieving people don't dwell on unpleasantness. They specialize
in positive memories. They prefer to make sunlight.
They practice letting go of destructive experiences.
Unsuccessful people handle unpleasantness in the opposite way. They dwell on the situation until they make it
a concrete memory. They won't free their minds of it,
and for days or weeks it's the last thing they think about
before they go to sleep.

Strange as it seems, the most important thing in your
life today isn't to lose weight. It is to become a person
who doesn't hoard anger, who doesn't handle difficulties
with a knife and fork. Weight loss will follow, won't it?
Say YES to that!

What have you done right today? You have seen how
anger easily spells danger. You have learned how to
handle anger as an achiever. Good for you!

**Today's Action Plan: I will not eat as a solution to
unpleasantness. I will practice making positive memories.**

Not Strictly from Hunger

Everything agitates me, and I experience every agitation as a sensation of hunger, even if I have just eaten.
Ellen West

We overeaters eat with our mouths and our feelings. Every situation and every emotion, negative and positive, is a cue for us to eat. Our response is to grab for our fork and knife. There is something robotic about such eating that indicates we are not aware of food as food. Food has become a reaction to every stimulus. Do you ever eat like a robot?

If overeaters eat in response to everything, what happens when our body sends us true hunger messages? We don't recognize them. That's the first adjustment most of us face when we begin to lose weight; we have to discern real hunger from emotional hunger.

When you are following a weight-losing plan and your body suddenly says, "Feed me now," you must look for the cause of the feeling. Are you just bored or upset? If you determine it's emotional hunger, work on the emotion. If it's real hunger, wait for the next meal. Say, "No, not now. I'll wait until mealtime." Say it out loud, right now. You could use the practice, couldn't you?

What have you done right today? You have recognized the difference between emotional and physical hunger. You have begun to teach your hunger patience.

Today's Action Plan: I will not eat because I'm bored or upset. I will lose pounds and gain patience.

Negative Attention

When you insist you're not the kind of person who can climb a mountain or make a speech, all you are saying is that up to now you haven't done it . . .
Mildred Newman and Bernard Berkowitz

You give yourself a lot of attention all right, negative attention. Every day you tell yourself that you are the "awfulest," "stupidest," "fattest" person in the world. You sell yourself short with such self-deprecation. It shows through in everything you do. Stop flaying yourself! Make peace within yourself. Do it today, won't you?

Start paying some positive attention to yourself. What are your fine points? Just by reading this book, you show that you want to change, you have the courage to face yourself, and you have the commitment to work for greater self-understanding. How many people do you know who are taking the same Action? Would you call them "awful," "stupid," or "fat?" No, you wouldn't!

You are a creator of solutions. You are giving yourself this chance today. Aim high. Aim for the top of a problem and start climbing. You should say YES to that, shouldn't you?

What have you done right today? You have learned how unjust it is to pay only negative attention to yourself. You realize it is finally time to be as fair to yourself as you are to others.

Today's Action Plan: I will not deprecate anything I am or do. I will pay only positive attention to myself.

Geared for Action

Instead of crying over spilt milk, go milk another cow.
                                                    Anonymous

The quotation above is an Action version of the "Don't cry over spilt milk" axiom, only it goes one important step further. "Don't cry" is passive, like "grin and bear it." This isn't good enough for overeaters. We must do something about this problem, not just lie down and accept it. Don't take it or leave it. You have choices. Now when problems arise, you gear for Action. That's the way you handle them, isn't it?

You are one who converts every problem into an opportunity. You must be, or else you'd be waiting for Lady Luck instead of reading this book. The door to a winning future is open to you. Walk right in.

Remind yourself every day that you are far better than you think you are. You don't need anyone to make you do what you know you should do. You know that you want to attain your natural weight, and you're learning how to do that. You have a mind, a factory fully equipped to work out your problems. You are a creator of solutions. There are no limits for you. Can you feel yourself day by day, month by month, growing in confidence? Say YES.

What have you done right today? There are so many things you are doing right. But today you reminded yourself you are a better person than you ever thought you were. Hooray for you!

Today's Action Plan: When problems arise, I will not cry over "spilt milk." I will go one important step further; I will get into Action to create new solutions.

Positive Concentration

Be not afraid of life. Believe that life is worth living, and
your belief will create the fact.

William James

Concentrate on the positive events of today. Burn negativity. Do you realize it is much easier to remember a happy experience than a sad one? You have to work hard to remember negative feelings. But your mind will readily cast aside the unpleasant if you cooperate. You're willing to at least consider this possibility, aren't you?

Think back to your childhood, to school days, to your first job. Your mind has a tendency to shrivel the unpleasant memories and give back a generalized rosy glow. Test yourself. Look at some old pictures taken at family gatherings. Your mind seems determined to cancel out any spat or unpleasantness. You tend to remember the happy times you had with friends and kin.

This is your mind's way of protecting you from negative memories. Your mind wants to cancel destructive ego experiences. Why don't you let it? Say YES to that. Now shout it.

What have you done right today? You found that your mind rejects unpleasant memories. Letting go of unpleasant memories is possible because your mind remembers only happiness.

Today's Action Plan: I will reject the negative. I will concentrate on the positive.

Conscience Power

*Every worthwhile accomplishment, big or little, has its
stages of drudgery and triumph; a beginning, a struggle,
and a victory.*

Anonymous

The second MindStep advises you to practice confidence
every day. One of the best ways to do this is to keep
your conscience clean. The power of your conscience is
enormous. It can lead you straight to your inevitable
victory over destructive eating. You'd be willing to do
just one thing today to harness this power, wouldn't
you?

Here it is: Do what you know is right for you. It's the
most practical suggestion you'll ever hear.

"How does that kind of advice make me thin?" you
may ask. Simple. When you do what is right for you (in
particular, follow your eating plan and exercise for
weight loss) two marvelous things happen. One, your
self-confidence grows; and two, you rid yourself of guilt.
Nothing erodes self-confidence more than guilt feelings.
When you gain confidence, you'll feel other people
reflecting confidence back to you.

Do what you know is right and your confidence will
soar. You see that, don't you?

What have you done right today? You have mobilized
the power of your conscience to build confidence. You
have gotten rid of guilt by doing what is right for you.
See? It all fits together.

Today's Action Plan: I will keep my conscience clean
and powerful. If I slip, I will immediately return to my
right way, so guilt won't make me eat.

Exercise Should Be Fun

I tried different kinds of exercise, hated them all, couldn't stick to one for more than a few days. Then I discovered aerobic dancing, something I really enjoyed. What a difference it has made in my weight and health!
A slender woman to her diet group

The woman quoted above started with a typical over-weight's attitude: if exercise is good for you, you won't like it. Do you approach exercise with the idea that, like grandmother's mustard plaster, it should hurt and be unpleasant if it's going to work? If that's the way you think, you'd be interested in a positive new way of thinking about exercise, wouldn't you?

You should love the exercise you do. Of course, you're going to love the results. The happy payoff is an energized body, sharp mind, vented frustrations, and best of all, burned-off fat. But the best way to get these results is for exercise to be fun. Unless it's fun, only a few utterly determined overeaters can stick to it long enough to be rewarded.

Create positive exercise experiences, ones you will look forward to every day. Try everything — aerobic dance, swimming, jogging, bicycling, walking, any combination of these, or some other aerobic exercise altogether. Which exercise did you love? Do it again, won't you?

What have you done right today? You have explored a startling new idea. Exercise should be one of the most enjoyable things you do each day.

Today's Action Plan: I will discover the exercises that are most fun for me to do. I will do them.

A New Way to Climb Off that Plateau

I hit a weight plateau, got discouraged, and slipped off the program. I felt as if I just couldn't cut my calories any lower.
                                        Overheard at a diet group

While losing weight, there comes the time when the body temporarily stops losing pounds. You're still doing what you should, yet your plan no longer seems to work. This is definitely a danger period. As a matter of fact, a weight plateau can be discouraging enough to send us back to the pain of overeating. You don't want this to happen to you, do you?

The usual advice to people on plateaus is, wait it out until you start losing again, or cut your caloric intake even more. As solutions, these are discouraging, aren't they?

Try this. Instead of grinning and bearing it or calorie-cutting, why not double your exercise? If you are exercising twenty minutes morning and evening, exercise forty minutes each time. By increasing your oxygen delivery rate, your body will begin to burn fat more efficiently and you'll be off that miserable plateau in no time.

There's more. Not only will you begin to lose weight again, but you'll improve strength and flexibility which makes it easier for you to exercise. See what a marvelous cycle you can create?

What have you done right today? Instead of giving up, you found a new solution for beating the plateau blahs. Know something? You can always do more than you think you can!

Today's Action Plan: I will create an exercise solution for the plateau problem. I will increase my exercise time.

June 12

Do You Wanna Dance?

*I love to dance, but my husband doesn't. Dance aerobics
is the perfect exercise for me.*
Overheard at dance exercise class

Exercise can fill more than one empty spot in your life. If
you want to dance and you don't have Fred Astaire or
Ginger Rogers for a partner, a dance class can be your
personal exercise and fulfill your terpsichorean fantasy as
well. Again, the point is to find an exercise that you like
for itself, not just because it's something you must do.
You understand the psychology behind this, don't you?

It makes good sense. Something you love to do, you
do more often, for longer periods, and with a great deal
more enthusiasm. The benefits will increase too. Did you
know that the more intense the exercise experience, the
more your right (or creative) side of the brain becomes
dominant? If you exercise for more than forty minutes at
a strenuous pace, your body releases natural opiates,
called endorphins, which give you a tremendous lift.

Today you're on the exercise fast track. You have a
deeper sense of security, knowing that you have the
stamina and strength to do anything you want. You
have a right to be strong and proud, don't you?

What have you done right today? You discovered that
you and exercise are perfect partners. May you live
happily together forever after!

**Today's Action Plan: I will make fitness my top
priority. I will elect exercise to be a partner in life.**

Mrs. Fantastic

Enthusiasm: It is nothing more nor less than faith in action.

Henry Chester

The tour bus traveled across the bleak, treeless Outer Hebrides landscape. All the sightseers were bored but one. "This is fantastic," the woman repeated, as she snapped pictures and exclaimed delightedly over each scrubby field of heather. Amused, her fellow passengers stared unbelievingly. The woman must be mad! She was obviously enjoying herself. But how? She had little reason to be so happy. Have you ever met someone with this much enthusiasm?

At the end of the bus ride, a curious passenger approached Mrs. Fantastic (by this time everyone called her that). "Thank you for making the trip more enjoyable for everyone," he said. "But don't tell me an experienced traveler like you really enjoyed that ride!" Smiling, she answered, "I certainly did. I learned something long ago when I started in the theater. A good actress doesn't just play a part, she lives it. I also remember playing a character who burst onto the stage, shouting, 'I've got good news!' I had the complete attention of that audience." Her eyes twinkled. "You see, my act still works."

Be a good news person, an actor if necessary. You will develop enthusiasm in yourself and in others, which comes right back to you. Get the enthusiasm habit, won't you?

What have you done right today? You have seen how good news people make their own lives — and the lives of all those around them — brighter. You want to make some sunshine.

Today's Action Plan: I will be enthusiastic wherever I am, whatever I do. I will be a good news person.

June 14

What Do You Want from Food?

Keep no secrets of thyself from thyself.
Greek Proverb

Socrates said that the unexamined life is not worth living. This wise observation is worth heeding. But we overweights avoid one particular examination because it's too painful, too frightening to face. The question: What do we want from food? The answer: We overeat because of feelings, as if food, especially sweets, held answers to our human loneliness. Yes, it's true, we turn to food when we need companionship, comfort, reassurance, or a sense of well-being.

Examine how you use food. Some people overeat to quiet emotional need. Ask yourself: What cookie gives me affection? What piece of cake puts its arms around me and says, "Well done"? What chocolate bar whispers, "I love you"?

Food can't substitute for human contact. Sure, you're taking a chance that another may not return the love or friendship you offer, but it's a risk worth taking. Food never gives you the emotional response you need. Overeating adds pounds and misery to your life, not affection or friendship.

Decide to risk human relationships. They may not always work out, but they won't add to your weight problem. You will believe that, won't you?

What have you done right today? You faced the important question: "What do I want from food?" You realize that food cannot give you the emotional support that will help you be thin. Right-eating, exercise, and Action MindStep attitudes can.

Today's Action Plan: I will examine my use of food. I will not try to satisfy my emotions with food.

Success Enemy Number One

Fear is the darkroom where negatives are developed.
Anonymous

The fears — of saber-toothed tigers or bands of hostile cave dwellers — that pumped adrenalin into the veins of our ancestors are gone. Today's everyday fears — of failure, embarrassment, loneliness, unhappy relationships — are likely to be based on emotional rather than physical survival. But whatever their roots, fears stop you from grasping at opportunities. They wear you down physically. Fear may even shorten your life. Did you know fear brings on hunger? That's right. It tricks us into thinking our physical letdown after an adrenalin rush is hunger, and we eat. Fear can be a powerful, negative force. You'd agree with that, wouldn't you?

Fear, manifested in anxiety or panic or worry, can mean a lack of confidence in yourself. But you can develop confidence. Nobody's born with confidence. It's learned by getting into Action. Postponing Action encourages fear while Action cures fear. And for every fear, there's a specific Action to take. If you fear doing something, do it; otherwise, you avoid it with one binge after another.

Fear is for losers. Action is for take-charge winners. You can remember that easily, can't you?

What have you done right today? You have learned that fear saps energy and increases hunger feelings. You have decided to get the Action habit and defeat your fears.

Today's Action Plan: I will not attempt to solve fear by overeating. I will face each fear with its Action solution.

Don't Resign Yourself to Fat

*If we want a thing badly enough, we can make it
happen. If we let ourselves be discouraged, that is proof
that our wanting was inadequate.*
                                            Dorothy L. Sayers

Have you ever thought, "Like it or not, I'll just have to
learn to live with this weight. I can't lose these excess
pounds. Mature, intelligent people accept the inevitable
and quit." That sounds reasonable, doesn't it? It's pure
rubbish!

Don't resign yourself to a fat life. No matter what
happened in the past, you'll never again accept being
depressed and feeling second-rate because of your
weight. You deserve the best, so get into Action. Want
to fulfill your desires. Want life to deliver good things.
Want success. These are all winner's wants.

Defeat disbelief by believing you can achieve whatever
you want. Don't tolerate the intolerable. Use your
intelligence by putting your desires into Action. Having
this book in your hands this minute is a good start. You
are determined to keep your desire for a high-energy life
at peak level. Set up a chain of longing that will never
break. You won't ever give up, will you?

What have you done right today? You have chosen
never to resign yourself to an unhappy, unproductive,
immobilized life. Congratulations, you made a wise
decision.

Today's Action Plan: I will think myself worthy of my
greatest desires. I will act rather than resign myself.

You're All Right

The important thing is not where you were or where you are but where you want to get.
Dave Mahoney

The first Action MindStep says that you have a unique worth. This means that you and you alone are in charge of your "all rightness." Do you understand? No matter what negative thing happens to you, even if someone says something terrible to you, you are still uniquely worthy. If you don't receive praise, don't get a raise, don't win the man/woman you want, there's nothing wrong with you. You are a special, worthy individual, and you are no longer dependent on outside influences for your sense of personal value, are you?

Sometimes we give other people permission to criticize us. Don't play that game. Too often we are easily hurt. Here's an effective solution to handling the criticism of others: don't spend one minute apologizing for your life to others.

And don't play the If Only game: if only it weren't for (job, mate, family, money), I could lose weight. You are the sum total of your own choices. You own them all. You are responsible, not dependent. When one of your choices proves to be a negative one, you see clearly what needs to be done, and you do it. Is this how you see yourself? You should.

What have you done right today? You have learned that your "all rightness" does not need validation from anyone but you. You are developing a solid understanding of your unique worth. It's yours, forever.

Today's Action Plan: I will be "all right" no matter what happens. I will be responsible, never apologizing, for my life.

The Ten Percent Solution

*The less one has to do, the less time
one finds to do it in.*

Lord Chesterfield

There's an old axiom: If you want something done, ask the busiest person you know. Such a person is one of the achievers. Busy people know how to organize their time and always seem to be able to take on just a little bit more. You can be that kind of person. Increase whatever you do by 10 percent, and soon you'll have a deserved reputation as a doer. You'd like to be known as a doer, wouldn't you?

You're better at everything than you think. There isn't one thing that you are doing in your life right now that you couldn't do better. You could increase your exercise time by 10 percent. If you now exercise a half-hour twice a day, 10 percent is only six more minutes per day. But over a month's time that's an increase of three hours, which would make a difference in your fitness and weight loss. Ten percent more daily exercise may seem like a trifle, but it adds up to as much as 20 more pounds lost per year. That's significant!

Or, instead of strolling down the street, walk 10 percent faster. You get more exercise, you arrive earlier, and there's something about walking faster that builds your self-confidence. (Experts say that muggers avoid people who walk with a fast, purposeful stride. Such people are more apt to defend themselves.) Wouldn't you like to push against the old limits? Ten percent more. That's all.

What have you done right today? You now know that you can ask more of yourself than you thought. It's a good feeling to know that, isn't it?

Today's Action Plan: I will be a 10 percenter. I will become 10 percent better at everything I do.

Stress Solution

Most of today's stress problems require a behavioral solution, not a physical one.

Dr. Herbert Benson

Most of us lead a pressure-cooker existence. Traffic jams, job-related anxiety, changing sex roles — all combine to jangle our nerves and tense our muscles. Too often an overweight's answer to stress is overeating, a physical response instead of a simple behavior change. Eating because of stress is a Catch-22 situation. It only piles on more stress. You'd like to get out of the stress-eat-stress cycle, wouldn't you?

Breathe slower. That's right. Remember the last time you were really stressed? Your breathing was rapid and shallow. This is time to apply the brakes. A breathing slow-down is an excellent two-minute cure for stress. Just begin a seven-second breath-in, breath-out cycle. Concentrate. Repeat this eight times, and in about two minutes stress is gone.

You see the difference, don't you? You won't be heaping overeating stress on top of what you already have. Try this small change in behavior. You can do it anywhere, anytime. *Do it.*

You are a problem-solver, you're activated, and that's exactly the way you've always wanted to be, isn't it?

What have you done right today? You learned a behavioral solution for everyday stress. You see that there are constructive ways to solve problems, which means you never need to turn to overeating again.

Today's Action Plan: I will seek non-food solutions to life's stresses. I will be a problem-solver.

The No-limit Life

My duty, as an intellectual, is to think, to think without restriction, even at the risk of blundering. I must set no limits within myself, and I must let no limits be set for me.

Jean-Paul Sartre

Dream no small dreams. Small dreams limit your imagination. Great dreams recognize no limits. This book teaches you how to throw off the limitation of excess weight. It says, go after that job, play that sport, join that club, dance, laugh, live. It says you have used only a fraction of your abilities. There is so much that you have, so much that makes you unique. You see that by now, don't you?

Your new life — the life of controlled eating, exercise, and take-charge attitudes — is not a struggle, but a cooperation with life. Before you got into Action, over-eating brought you into conflict with your own intelligence, triggering struggle and self-disgust. Those days are gone forever.

Great dreamers set no inner limits and recognize no outer limits. They move. They know that the harder they go, the closer they come to achievement. Isn't that what you're after, achievement of your dreams? Say YES to that, won't you?

What have you done right today? You have prepared yourself to dream great dreams, and to put them into Action quickly. You are a mover, unlimited and undaunted. With that kind of winning attitude, you can't miss!

Today's Action Plan: I will allow no limits within or without myself. I will get into Action and cooperate with life.

June 21

Three Excuses (All Wrong) for Not Exercising

"After a long day at work, I don't have the energy to exercise." "I get enough exercise around the house." "Exercising only makes me hungrier."
Results of Harris Poll

This book keeps hammering away at the theme that exercise is one key to permanent weight loss. So if you're not exercising, you must have an excuse, a good excuse. Is it one of the three popular excuses offered by polled adults who don't exercise?

"After a long day on the job, I don't have any energy left." Is that your excuse? Wrong! When you're de-energized, that's the time you need to exercise most. Remain inactive and you spend your evening exhausted. Exercise gives energy!

"I get enough exercise around the house/job/school." Is that your excuse? Wrong again! You may work hard, stopping and starting dozens of times, but few jobs give you the sustained aerobic exercise you need for your health.

"Exercise makes me hungrier; I'll start eating more and gain weight." Is that your excuse? Still wrong! Exercise is an appetite suppressant. You'll eat less food after you exercise, and your body will burn more calories.

If you are an exercise holdout, add exercise to your diet menu today. Find three good excuses to exercise. Try these. "I'll burn more calories." "I'll feel better." "I'll look better." Of course, you want all that. Then you have three great excuses to start exercising, don't you?

What have you done right today? You heard three bad excuses not to exercise and saw right through them. You found three smart reasons to exercise and decided these are good excuses for you. Get moving!

Today's Action Plan: I will be fit. I will treat my body like a muscle born to be worked.

Dr. Right

Doctors have laughed at me, scolded me, and refused to treat me if I didn't lose weight.

Overheard at a diet club

You have a right to the best medical care available. Are you getting it? At a diet group meeting, one woman said, "No matter what I go to the doctor for — flu, ingrown toenail, infection — he blames it on my weight." Another woman added, "I've been humiliated so many times that I don't go to my doctor even when I should." How do you feel about the medical treatment you get?

If any doctor you consult for medical help treats you in less than a dignified manner, fire him or her. You simply don't have to take less than the best professional treatment available. You may very well want your doctor to guide you on certain parts of your weight program, but that's your decision to make or to change anytime you wish. You're in charge. Remember that.

If you're unhappy with your present physician, seek out another. There is a doctor right for you. Doctor Right will be supportive of your efforts, optimistic about your new program, and will never bully you. And you won't permit the doctor's staff to use derogatory language about your size. No. Never.

In every way, you have taken charge of your health and your life. If your doctor doesn't live up to your expectations, you change doctors, don't you?

What have you done right today? You have a new self-respect. From now on, you will expect dignified and attentive service from your physician and the medical staff.

Today's Action Plan: I will be self-respectful and demand the same from the professionals I pay. I will have the medical help I need and deserve.

Become a Now Person

It is vain to say human beings ought to be satisfied with tranquillity; they must have action, and they will make it if they cannot find it.

Charlotte Brontë

"I'll start tomorrow/Monday/next week/January 1." When you postpone weight-losing Action with these tomorrow promises, you are implying that conditions will be better at some special future time. But when that time arrives, conditions usually aren't better. Conditions are never perfect. They never will be. Now is all you ever have to use, whatever the conditions. Don't you agree?

Be a doer, not a procrastinator; an optimist, not a pessimist. You have an idea of what you want your life to be. Do you know that all of your life's accomplishments come from an idea you acted on? If you don't like your life, you can change it. Right now.

This is the best time you own. Learn to think in terms of this minute, hour, and day. Be an I'm-beginning-now person. Be an I-can't-wait-to-start-my-new-life person. Act alive!

You are perfectly capable of putting together the best program for your life, capable of achieving it, and capable of living with your achievement. Success is an idea you'd like to act on, isn't it?

What have you done right today? You see that you will be satisfied with nothing less than Action. You learned that you have the capacity to become a doer and an optimist. You feel alive!

Today's Action Plan: I will make today's conditions just right for Action. I will be a can't-wait-to-start person.

Soaring Goals

The spirit that does not soar is destined to grovel.
Benjamin Disraeli

The world is moving. If you don't move with it, it will leave you behind. The way to keep pace is to set goals, not just I-wish-I-could goals. They aren't goals. "I'm going to lose X number of pounds, get down to my natural weight, become physically fit, and win success in my life." Now *there* are some goals! They give you a definite idea of where you want to go. You're ready to press ahead, aren't you?

Ten years hence seems far away as you read this, but before you know it, it will pass. Where do you want to be ten years from today? What do you want to accomplish on the job, at home, in your social life? What do you want to look like? Write it down. Now read what you've written. You have written a plan of Action. Now you have a ten-year plan of Action.

To make your ten-year plan a reality, begin to set smaller goals. Count each small goal as a step toward winning. These efforts pay off. It's the best idea you'll hear today.

Setting and achieving personal goals is one of the greatest joys in living. That's right, isn't it?

What have you done right today? You looked at the next decade and took charge of where you want to be. It's going to be a great ten years!

Today's Action Plan: I will soar into the rest of my life by making a ten-year plan. I'll decide where and what I want to be, and set the goals to get me there.

How Do You Rate?

Our deeds determine us, as much as we determine our deeds.

George Eliot

Today, as you approach this year's halfway mark, is a good time to review and rate the past months. Naturally, the first evaluation an overweight makes is, "How much weight did I lose?" That's a legitimate question. But you should ask another one too: "How many small goals did I reach on the way to my ultimate goal?" Overall progress, while important, isn't nearly as important as the direction you're heading. You're moving step by step, goal by goal toward success, aren't you?

What does the word "success" mean to you? Without doubt it means controlled eating, a fit body, and a take-charge attitude. Those are fantastic goals, worthy of you, and isn't your life definitely happier?

Of course, you still have problems. Don't expect unrealistic perfection from yourself or your life. Expect that you will continue to change. Be open to it. Expect that others will not be able to fulfill you. Be ready to fulfill yourself. Expect that others will not be responsible for you. Own yourself.

As you grow in confidence, you will feel more and more that you have embarked on a rewarding relationship with yourself. As the months pass, it will evolve into a caring, trusting companionship based on self-regard and winning attitudes. You are one of the really fortunate people of this world, aren't you?

What have you done right today? You evaluated your performance and reaffirmed your resolve to take charge of the food in your life. That is a great deal for one day.

Today's Action Plan: I will renew my commitment to success. Today I will move one small goal closer to my desired body.

This Is the Day

SEIZE THIS DAY! Begin now! Each day is a new life.
Seize it. Live it. For in today already walks tomorrow.
David Guy Powers

Isn't it amazing how we take the numbers on the calendar for granted? Do you think they're just marks on paper, 365 number combinations for the twelve months? These numbers are codes for your brain to turn into ideas, desires, and meanings. Each day is a miracle waiting to happen to you. Let your brain decode positive meanings for this day, won't you?

This is the day that will give you new life. Seize it! It is real. So many ideas in life are invisible, leaving no footprints. This day will leave a footprint on your life. This day you will not accept the number 26 on the calendar as just another mark on paper. No, today will be a day that will leave a mark on your life. Each day these marks are added together. Now you are moving toward a life of achievement, a life of victory over food.

Today. Seize it! It is yours. It is the most precious of your possessions. No one can take it from you. It can be thrown away, but it is unstealable. And these twenty-four hours are given the same, neither more nor less, to every other human. You're going to use the wonderful gift of today, aren't you? Say YES.

What have you done right today? Of all the right things you have done today, the most right is your commitment to make this day, and each day of your life, well-lived. That's a rare gift you've given yourself.

Today's Action Plan: I will seize this day. I will make this day count in some special way.

Facing It

I nearly died in the supermarket when a little boy said in a loud voice, "Mommy, what makes people fat?" I didn't turn around; I knew he was pointing at me.

A TOPS member

Does every criticism from others throw you into a defensive position? Are you depressed for days? The only cure for defensiveness over what other people say is to be safe in the knowledge of the changes you're making in your life. You know who you are and where you're going. Soon others will see and know it too, won't they?

You don't have to own cruel remarks based on your size. That you never have to do. And don't feel that every mention of weight (or anything derogatory you overhear) is aimed at you. Beware of rabbit ears! This sports term refers to a competitor who hears every little negative comment from the stands, and as a result, loses winning concentration.

When you are accomplishing what you know you want to accomplish in your life, your mind is at peace. Conflict and guilt are absent. Your mind is positive and is drawn to the positive. You may overhear negative things, but they don't touch you, they don't belong to you.

The beauty of your new life is your discovery that you are greater than you thought, than anyone thought. That's true, isn't it?

What have you done right today? You know that you are too self-respectful to accept any abusive remarks seriously. Your new positive outlook attracts constructive comment and sheds the negative.

Today's Action Plan: I will disown any cruel remarks based on my size. Instead, I will concentrate on maintaining the positive attitude that will bring me a thinner body and happier life.

June 28

The Best Way to Beat Pressure

Everything comes to him who hustles while he waits.
Thomas A. Edison

Pressure, from outside and inside, is a part of our times. We try to do our very best, hoping others will take notice and be pleased. A mother makes a school costume and wonders if her daughter will like it. Business people strive for that big promotion. Children take school exams and worry that they may not pass. We all hope we'll come through the crucial moment, don't we?

The important thing in any pressure situation is not to overeat while awaiting the outcome. Successful authors learn, as a matter of self-preservation, that once they mail a precious manuscript to a publisher, they must hustle right on to a new book. If a rejection notice comes, so be it; they're so immersed in the new project that the turn-down doesn't hurt nearly as much.

Hustle while you wait. When you do a piece of good work, don't wait for the applause. It may come. On the other hand, your job may be ignored or get no satisfactory response. If you sit around expectantly waiting for praise, you'll be crushed if you don't get it, and this is sure to sabotage your morale and kill your incentive. But if you've moved on to something new and interesting, you're not apt to get bogged down in self-pity.

Make accomplishing the job the most important thing. Then get going on the next job, won't you?

What have you done right today? You've learned to get on with your job, eating right for weight loss, exercising for a beautifully fit body, and constructing positive attitudes. That takes a lot of hustle, but you've got it.

Today's Action Plan: I won't lock my life into a holding pattern during a pressure situation. I will do my job, and then hustle on.

Pressure Well-met

As exercise strengthens the body, pressure well-met strengthens the spirit. Without its occasional discipline, character suffers.

Ira Wolff

When you're under pressure — starting a new job, moving to a new home, any major life change — don't use food as a pressure safety valve. Overeating might give the illusion of control, but it's only an illusion. Soon overeating will take its toll, ravaging your self-esteem, leaving your body and mind weaker. There is a happier alternative. When pressure builds, there is no better release than physical exercise. It's essential. Your mind is distracted when your body is engaged. Exercise is the most complete and positive form of escape from pressure. Haven't you found it so?

Pressure well met, whether by exercise or attitude, simply means pressure well used. Whenever you are under pressure, you have a unique opportunity to do something, and to be good at it. Wherever there is pressure, there is a challenge. When an Olympic athlete crosses the finish line, reporters never ask, "How could you do that under pressure?" They know that pressure is essential to winners; it's the kick in the pants that helps them get to the top. Pressure causes you to concentrate your energy completely.

Today your safety valve for pressure comes from right-eating, exercise, and your new take-charge attitude. Concentrate on these and win, won't you?

What have you done right today? You learned that overeating is only an illusion of control. You chose to conquer overeating by using pressure as a challenge.

Today's Action Plan: I will use pressure to help me concentrate on my goals. I will concentrate on winning.

What's to Become of You?

You will become as small as your controlling desire; as great as your dominant aspiration.

James Allen

Suppose you're the boss and you are offered two people: one who has great talent, but is a pessimist; another with average ability, but who bubbles with enthusiasm. Which one would you hire? You'd do well to employ the second person because enthusiasm is tenacious and gets the job done. Enthusiasm gives birth to endurance, whereas pessimism kills it. Over the long pull, talent will not get you as far as persistence. You believe that, don't you?

Don't bother with little wishes. What is your dominant desire? Name it, and begin working for it. Any day is a good day to start.

You have one great aspiration, don't you? It is to take charge of each day to shake your food dependency. Overeating made your life a shambles. Now you've rejected excess food as a way to manage your life.

You have a job to do. To do it you need all the enthusiasm and persistence you can summon. Keep your mind on achieving a thinner winner's life; stay too busy to be unsure; keep looking for the best within you, and finding it. Believe that. Enthusiasm is belief which caught fire! That's right, isn't it? Say YES.

What have you done right today? You see that enthusiasm fired by belief in yourself will help you reach your life goal. You are becoming the kind of person everyone admires. It's exciting to know you!

Today's Action Plan: I will pursue my goals enthusiastically. I will work the Twelve Action MindSteps persistently.

A Small Beginning

*It matters not how small the beginning may seem to be;
what is once well done is done forever.*
Henry David Thoreau

If you just started this book, you did so because your life
hasn't been what you wanted it to be. We all have basic
wants: security, health, comfort, confidence, a wish to
be admired, and a desire for self-improvement. Overeating and the resultant overweight strikes at every basic
human need. Is it any wonder your overeating produces
such anxiety?

The most important thing for you to do is to make a
beginning, right now, no matter how overweight you
are. You may have thought that life passed you by, that
there was no hope for you. Banish such silly thoughts
from your mind! Listen. Today your heart will beat
103,680 times, you'll breathe 23,040 times, and you'll
speak 4,800 words. Make every beat, breath, and word
count as a beginning toward your winning life!

During the days to come you'll learn about the Twelve
Action MindSteps, guides to a wonderful life. (If you
have been reading this book for some time, now is an
excellent time to review those vital steps.) Get ready. Get
set. Now go! You see all the possibilities, don't you?

What have you done right today? By reading this
page, you show your willingness to turn your life
around. You opened your mind to a new way to achieve
your basic needs.

**Today's Action Plan: I will make a small beginning
well done by improving my weight-loss eating plan.
With every heartbeat, breath, word, I will make today
work.**

July 2

Overcoming Despair

The darkest hour is only sixty minutes.
Author unknown

Did you overeat recently? Physically, did you feel logy, headachey, hung over? Emotionally, did you feel ashamed, disgusted, despairing? "Why?" you ask yourself. "Why did I do that?" You overate because overeating was your idea for trying to make life more comfortable, but it's a bad idea. It's time to get a better coping solution than overeating. You see that, don't you?

You used overeating as a way to cope with life because you had trouble "imagineering." Imagineering is a way to overcome the despair of the overeating trap. Try picturing the person you want to become, then dream his or her dream. Visualize the healthy, attractive body within your present body. Dwell on this vision. See the firm skin drawn taut around your chin, upper arms, and thighs. See your muscle-firmed abdomen and buttocks.

Concentrate. Imagine yourself exactly the way you want to be. Isn't that a pretty picture? It's a better idea, any day, than overeating. So do it, won't you? Say YES, and mean it with all your heart.

What have you done right today? You see that your darkest hour of overeating can be changed to a bright new idea of self-imagining. You know that you can achieve what you want by dreaming a greater dream, and then seeing yourself in it. Dream on!

Today's Action Plan: I will get rid of overeating as an idea that doesn't work. Instead, I will imagine my body as I want it to be, which will help me reach my goal.

July 3

Get the Review Habit

*There is only one success . . . to be able to spend your
life in your own way.*
Christopher Morley

During this month, you'll be reviewing the Twelve
Action MindSteps. These principles of thought and
Action form the bedrock of this book. Review is repetition. As with anything you really want to learn, you
must review the MindSteps often — daily at first — until
you make them as much a habit as your old destructive
behavior. Then there is the Action kind of repetition.
Repeat a good, new Action often enough, and you will
create a nice new habit and erase a bad one. You can
agree so far, can't you?

Life is meant to be a glorious adventure. When you
are prepared, every moment glows with new possibilities. As you go beyond the thought process and put your
thinking into Action, life can be a marvelous challenge.
Certainly, as long as you are actively engaged in working the MindSteps, you are not overeating. Why?
Because it's impossible to raise your self-esteem and do
the thing you despise.

Each of the Twelve Action MindSteps has a simple
message: you are worthy of your love and care. Accept
this month of review as an opportunity to know yourself
better and to grow in self-love. If you do, you can begin
to live life your own way. You see that, don't you?

What have you done right today? You recognize the
need to review and repeat the Twelve Action MindSteps
until you make them part of you.

**Today's Action Plan: I will review the MindSteps until
they are part of me. I will grow in self-worth.**

The First Action MindStep

*Granted that it is difficult . . . to be sure exactly who
you are, and granted also that there is a sense in which
every person ought to live as if they were on the way to
becoming a different person . . . the truth remains that
all mental and spiritual health begins
with self-acceptance.*

Samuel Butler

Some discouraged overweights find it difficult to believe
that they are indeed worthy people. Yet to achieve the
weight loss they seek, it is essential that they achieve self-
acceptance — come to an acknowledgment, even a
supreme consciousness — of self-worth. That is why
Action MindStep number one says: **Develop a solid
understanding of your unique worth.** You can work on
that, can't you?

Perhaps you said, "I want to, but . . . ." You added
the "but" because you felt helpless. You believed you
were too weak to take Action to get out of a rut. You're
wrong.

Want to save yourself enough to make the Twelve
Action MindSteps happen to you. Make such a want
your Action for today. Positive Action halts any lurking
"I can'ts."

Begin your Action. You will gain an immediate sense
of worth if you devote time right now to your well-
being. Believe that you are worthy, won't you? Say YES
and take Action.

What have you done right today? You accepted the
idea of your unique worth and you determined to earn
even greater confidence and strength by getting into
Action.

**Today's Action Plan: I will stop the flow of "I can'ts."
I will eat as I know I should, so that I will be able to
accept and understand my unique worth.**

Imagineering

*When the will and the imagination are antagonistic, it is
always the imagination which wins,
without any exception.*

Emile Coué

It's an old trick. Concentrate all the sun's energy through
a glass onto a pile of twigs and you'll start a fire.
Likewise, if you can concentrate your imagination on
one goal, you will ignite your wishes into a flame of
Action. The secret is to concentrate all your imagination
on what you want most. You can do that, can't you?

Imagine the body you want, the one that already
exists within you. Imagine that your inner body is
visible. See it! Feel it! Concentrate all your imaginative
power on it. (Your concentrated imagination is infinitely
more powerful than when it is scattered among a whole
shopping list of wants.) One desire, a new body. Now
concentrate!

"Imagineering" is simply giving a pictured form to
your goal. It is a powerful way of giving substance to
your wishes and thereby making them happen. Stop
right here and concentrate on the thin person inside
yourself, won't you?

What have you done right today? You determined to
focus all your imaginative energy on one desire, the look
and feel of your new body. Each day you can concentrate on one goal until you have imagineered a whole
new winning life.

Today's Action Plan: I will concentrate all my imagination on my beautiful, hidden, inner body to make it
visible. I will be an imaginative doer.

July 6

The Second Action MindStep

Keep on doing what it took to get started.
John L. McCaffrey

Practice makes perfect, right? The second Action Mind-Step says: **Practice confidence every day.** Can you actually develop confidence in yourself by practicing it? You bet you can. And with an emerging confidence in yourself, you will whip your weight problem. From now on, you're going to act as if you had confidence to spare. Don't you agree that life will be more fun when you face it with a confident spirit?

Indecision is a killer. It saps your emotional strength. It pits your positive and negative selves against each other. Indecision laughs at your goals and tangles you in confusion. Confidence, on the other hand, expects — even demands — that you achieve and win. Now do you see why you need to practice confidence?

Nothing builds your confidence faster than achieving small goals right away and every day. So get into Action. Make your goal for today eating right for a weight loss. How much weight you lose is important, but even more important, you set the small goal of right-eating for one day, and you did it. What a confidence builder! Make a habit of confidently setting and achieving this small goal each day. Soon you'll be able to do more and set other goals. Speak confidently about what you're doing. Use phrases like, "I'll take the initiative." "I'll swing into Action." "Let's go!" There's no stopping you, is there?

What have you done right today? You see that indecision is the killer of dreams. You have replaced indecision with a thinning, winning confidence.

Today's Action Plan: I will speak, think, and act confidently. I will practice confidence by achieving a minimum of one small goal a day.

You Have a Good Thing

He that labors in any great or laudable undertaking has his fatigues first supported by hope and afterward rewarded by joy.

Dr. Samuel Johnson

You've heard the old saying, "Where there is life, there is hope." Forget it. It's backwards. Actually, where there is hope there is life. There is no life without hope. When you read these pages you prove that you are alive and hopeful. That's a good thing, isn't it?

Hope helps you imagine how it will feel when you look in the mirror and see your new, vibrant, attractive body. Hope helps you dream, set and make goals.

Hope is an essential part of the good beginning you make every day. It will lift you out of the overeater's shadow of despair into the sunshine of the winner's circle.

Ponder this question. What one thing would you do if you knew you could not fail? You can begin doing it right now. You cancel overeater's despair with hope. Bank on hope, won't you?

What have you done right today? You have traded your shackled existence for a life filled with hope. You know that hope and Action will lead straight to joy.

Today's Action Plan: I will put hope first so that I can live. Today I will take Action and do what I want most in this world.

*

The Third Action MindStep

*Nothing is a greater impediment to being on good terms
with others than being ill at ease with yourself.*
                                        Honoré de Balzac

The third Action MindStep says: **Radiate warmth.** Your
caring warmth should flow in two directions: out to
others, and in to your deepest self. Forgive yourself for
overeating and you can then forgive anyone anything.
Being overweight in a thin-is-right society is enough of a
burden, but suffering without warmth and self-caring is
downright unbearable. There is no magic formula for
creating enough warmth for yourself and others. As a
child you received warmth, thus learning to give it. As
an adult, the situation is reversed: you must give warmth
first, before you can receive it. You understand how
Action has to come before reward, don't you?

Loving yourself just as you are today, however imperfect, is like a discovery. It's like turning on an X-ray that
reveals the real you underneath the flesh. Self-love not
only gives you the capacity to care about others, it gives
you the strength and confidence to make changes in your
life.

This loving warmth is something you must acquire for
yourself. Strangely enough, gratitude seems to be the
spark that ignites your warmth. Cultivate an attitude of
gratitude for what you have, and, suddenly, what you
want is much more possible. You see how that could be,
don't you?

What have you done right today? You learned to
judge yourself with a caring heart. You see that you
create the darkness in your life when you stand in the
way of your own light.

**Today's Action Plan: I will radiate caring without and
within. I will be grateful that I have a plan for chasing
the shadows from my life.**

July 9

Your Focal Point

Happiness is the exercise of vital powers, along lines of
excellence, in a life affording them scope.
Edith Hamilton

Exercise your vital powers. That means that your life
should have a focal point to give it meaning. A life filled
with aimless rounds of meaningless activities dissipates
your vital powers. It tires and bores you. For an
overeater, lacking a goal is a catastrophe; food binges
are inevitable in an attempt to overwhelm the emptiness.
You can see that, can't you?

Every day you uncover talents and strive for excellence. Make today count. You don't have to make a
spectacular discovery, but you can make today a little
better than yesterday. The most satisfying way an
overeater can do this is to eat and exercise for physical
and mental fitness. Concentrate all your powers on this
point.

Today you'll accomplish things because of what you
are thinking right now. Positive thoughts will work for
you if you think they will; if you think they won't, they
won't. Go on, put the positive side of your mind to
work. It's right for you. That's so, isn't it?

What have you done right today? You learned the
importance of developing the right focus and using all
your power to reach it.

Today's Action Plan: I will focus all my energy on my
ultimate weight goal. I trust that what I read in these
pages will work for me.

The Fourth Action MindStep

*You may not realize it when it happens, but a kick in the
teeth may be the best thing in the world for you.*
Walt Disney

The fourth Action MindStep says: **Learn what your fears
are.** Why? Because fear is your principal enemy and
hides behind many disguises. The biggest fear you mask
is that you will not be able to withstand a kick in the
teeth. No matter how many times you fight back from
defeat, a negative critic inside you convinces you that
you are doomed to lose. Are you aware of your negative
critic?

When we overeaters don't recognize past courage and
therefore can't imagine ourselves acting courageously,
we're really practicing a kind of negative arithmetic. We
may have overcome adversity ten times in the past year.
But if only once we didn't, then we subtract one from
ten and get zero. That negative critic is a poor mathematician.

Fear is basically a lack of confidence in our future
behavior, and there's only one antidote for that: Action.
Fear tells you to be a quitter; it predicts you will fail and
fall. Self-confidence tells you that when you fight your
way through fear you can't fail, because even if you lose,
you learn. Then you can go on to win next time.

Here's some simple, positive arithmetic. One, learn
your fears. Two, inoculate yourself with the antidote for
fear, confidence. Three, head for the winner's circle. Do
it today, won't you?

What have you done right today? You made courage
count more than fear of failing. Since you see that you
learn from every mistake, there is no such thing as
failing.

Today's Action Plan: I will subtract one from ten and
get confidence. I will march ahead — one, two, three.

Be All Here

*There is one thing we can do, and the happiest people
are those who do it to the limit of their ability. We can
be completely present. We can be all here. We can . . .
give all our attention to the opportunity before us.*
                                        Mark Van Doren

Today is a great opportunity. Give all your attention to
the opportunity of this day. Forget yesterday and tomorrow. Be all here. Be completely in the now. Lock your
attention onto the opportunity this day presents to you.
Above all, want to be with yourself today, won't you?

We try to wiggle out and escape from the present for
just one reason, to be rid of ourselves. What folly! Self-
hate is spiritually unconstitutional. It's a cruelty that
breaks the laws of love and humanity.

Join the happy people now. Give all your attention to
the opportunity of this day. What is your opportunity?
To do what you know you want to do; to become a
little more what you want to be; and to gracefully move
your body, mind, and spirit further from the desire for
excess food. What a day to be all here! You see that,
don't you? Say YES with the happy people.

What have you done right today? You see today as a
great opportunity to be really present for yourself, to be
all here for you. You want to banish from this — your
day of opportunity — any imagined need to overeat.

**Today's Action Plan: I will be all here. Whatever
opportunity this day holds, I will seize it.**

The Fifth Action MindStep

*It is difficult to say what is impossible, for the dream of
yesterday is the hope of today
and the reality of tomorrow.*

Robert H. Goddard

The fifth Action MindStep says: **Acknowledge a burning
desire to be thin and healthy.** Sounds simple. Every
overweight has that desire every waking minute. The
key to this MindStep is the word "acknowledge." Overeat, and your unacknowledged desire can be drowned by
food. But acknowledge your desire to yourself, even to
the world, and it becomes so strong that it refuses to be
suppressed. That's right, isn't it?

Acknowledge your resolve that today you will not
overeat. You will do exactly what you want to do. You
may ask, "Doesn't that mean I'll overeat?" No. You
despise overeating! If you do exactly what you want to
do, you can't do what you despise.

What is tomorrow's reality? A life of freedom from
excess food and unwanted flesh, being creative, energized, physically and mentally fit. All this, because today
you have a burning desire to be thin and healthy.
Acknowledge your desire, won't you? Give it life.

What have you done right today? You see that to
suppress your burning desire to be thin is to risk
smothering it with extra food. You won't take that risk.

**Today's Action Plan: I will acknowledge, to myself
and others, that I have a powerful desire to be thin and
healthy. I will provide the desire to succeed.**

A Chris Evert-Lloyd She Isn't (but Who Cares?)

> *My friends thought I was crazy — tennis*
> *at my age and weight!*
>
> Woman at a tournament

Is there an exercise or sport that attracts you, but you're embarrassed to try? Listen to this California woman: "I was forty-nine years old and weighed 185 pounds when we moved to our new condo with nearby tennis courts," she said. "For the first few weeks, I stared at those courts wishing I was twenty-five and thin."

"One day while walking my dog," she went on, "I ran into the resident pro. Just to make light conversation, I said, 'I'd be one of your pupils if I were only twenty years younger and thirty pounds lighter' (I lied about the pounds). Ignoring my excuse, the pro offered me a complimentary lesson due new tenants. Something made me keep that appointment, even though I didn't have the proper clothes — it's hard to find tennis clothes in my size — and I had to borrow a racket."

Have you ever had a chance to try a sport you thought you'd love? Did you do it?

What happened to this shy court novice? Five years after her first lesson, this formerly fat woman weighs only 135 pounds and plays tournament tennis. "It wasn't easy to get out there," she says, "but I forced myself, and I'm happy I did. Now I feel stronger — both physically and emotionally." You'd like to have those feelings, wouldn't you?

What have you done right today? You have re-evaluated the sports and exercises that you were too timid to try. That's a wonderful move you've made!

Today's Action Plan: From this day on, I will not limit my exercise horizons. I will move more today than ever before — and keep moving.

The Sixth Action MindStep

*It is the artist's business to create sunshine
when the sun fails.*

Romain Rolland

You are the artist of your environment. When it rains on you, you don't have to wait for others to change the landscape. As the sixth Action MindStep says: **Make your own sunlight.** This MindStep isn't a witless let's-all-be-happy statement. It is a basic truth. You light your own way just as you cast your own dark shadows. You see that, don't you?

Even the happiest people have some darkness, but the life of overeaters seems especially somber. Self-loathing darkens their way. On the other hand, doing what you want for yourself can brighten your way.

The sixth MindStep, as do the other MindSteps, leads you in one direction, toward right-eating, physical and mental fitness, a thinner body, and a life of inner comfort. This achievement is exactly what you want and you will not be content without it. You instinctively know that such a life will light up your environment. The light of Action banishes the darkness of depression.

Color your world bright. Let the sunshine in, won't you?

What have you done right today? You learned that, like an artist, you control the light in your life. You see that by doing for yourself what you know you should, you paint your days with bright colors.

Today's Action Plan: I will paint my day from the bright end of my artist's palette. I will light my own way with good choices.

Beyond Feelings

*Doubt of any kind cannot be resolved
except by action.*

Thomas Carlyle

Every one of the MindSteps goes beyond feelings. Too many overeaters are immersed in self-awareness, mistakenly believing that learning about their emotional selves is Action in itself. Insight, even a significant behavioral one, is only action with a small "a." Such self-discoveries give us no more than a minor boost unless we use them to take effective charge of our lives. Effective — that's an interesting word, isn't it?

The dictionary defines "effective" as "producing the desired result." Is the way you're living now producing the result you desire?

Far too often, we overeaters settle for holding a little piece of life's emotional low ground. We have too many self-doubts to throw ourselves into the battle for the high ground of freedom from dependence on excess food.

Today you will go beyond feelings and doubt. Your desire to be physically and emotionally fit will power your courage to act. You will eat right, exercise, and get beyond feelings into Action. You are not content to hold your own. You choose to take effective charge of your life. That's right, isn't it? Say YES.

What have you done right today? You learned that being stuck at the feeling level is not Action. You know that when you take effective Action, you produce the results you want, a thinning-winning life.

Today's Action Plan: I will recognize Action by results. I will climb to the high ground of independence from food.

July 16

The Seventh Action MindStep

*We must have courage to bet on our ideas, to take the
calculated risk, and to act. Everyday living requires
courage if life is to . . . bring happiness.*
Maxwell Maltz

Take charge of your life, reads the seventh Action
MindStep. This basic idea is expressed other ways. If life
is a feast, be the host, not the guest. Or don't be a
passenger, be the driver. You get the idea, don't you?

The spice of life, contrary to the popular expression, is
not variety. The spice of life is choice. And the spiciest,
most successful life is an unending series of choices well
made. Making your own choices doesn't automatically
mean they will always be right, but right or wrong, the
choices that really work for you are the ones you make
for yourself.

This seems so clear. Yet surprisingly, many people
(thin ones, too) see themselves as powerless over their
own lives. They wait for someone to tell them what to
do next.

Success favors active, take-charge people — those who
have the courage to take risks and, above all, to act on
their own wants, enhance their probabilities of success
and happiness. Bet on yourself as a thinner winner
today, won't you?

What have you done right today? You decided that,
to get where you want to go, you're going to jump into
the driver's seat. That's the "rightest" decision you could
make this or any other day.

**Today's Action Plan: I will take charge and make my
own choices. I will make choices that take me closer to
independence from overeating.**

A Magnificent Obsession

The spending of our energies is the greatest possible stimulus to their recreation.

Charles Darwin

This is a true story. Ray, an overweight, middle-aged business executive, had all the trademarks of a compulsive personality, and his compulsion wasn't with food alone. He was a chain smoker, a workaholic, and he had a drinking problem as well. You recognize the compulsiveness, don't you?

But Ray had a real scare one day. While walking down a staircase he became dizzy and disoriented. His doctor told him what he already knew, that he was literally killing himself. The doctor urged him to quit overeating, smoking, and drinking, and to try regular exercise — jogging, perhaps?

Shaken by the doctor's dire warnings, Ray began to eat right, worked a program to quit smoking and drinking, and embarked on a jogging schedule. It was tough at first. After the first few steps he was gasping, and his rarely-used muscles ached. But the aches were good aches.

Ray's new love became an obsession. One mile increased to two, then to five. Now he's competing in marathons, and his time keeps getting faster.

Ray harnessed his compulsiveness into a healthy activity. Are you an overachiever of the wrong things? Can you channel your energies into a beneficial habit?

What have you done right today? You have learned that you can turn your compulsiveness to your own advantage successfully. This is inspiring, isn't it?

Today's Action Plan: I will look for an exercise to get healthfully "compulsive" about. I know that this habit will make me thinner.

The Eighth Action MindStep

Do not look back. It will neither give you back the past nor satisfy your daydreams. Your duty, your reward, your destiny are here and now.

Dag Hammarskjöld

Today is not just "the first day of the rest of your life." Today is more urgent. It's the only time that you have to work with now. But the eighth Action MindStep isn't concerned with time alone. It says: **Do whatever has to be done now.** That doesn't mean being busy for busy's sake. It's quite specific — do what you know you must do. You could miss the significance of this MindStep unless you study its meaning, couldn't you?

Today is a time to deliberately let go of unpleasant overeating memories. If you look back and find failure, regret, or self-deprecation following you, let those feelings go.

Move forward today toward the vitally interesting life you want. You aren't limited by yesterday. Everything in your world is fresh, joyful, creative, and fulfilling. Live fully in today. This minute, if you don't overeat, holds a reward which you can carry into the future. Minute-upon-minute of accomplishment is what you want so desperately from life, isn't it? Say, YES.

What have you done right today? You assimilated the dual message of the eighth Action MindStep: Do it now, and do whatever has to be done.

Today's Action Plan: I will not postpone any part of my take-charge program for a thinner life. I will act now.

July 19

Motion Equals Emotion

Remember, motions are the precursors of emotions. You can't control the latter directly, but only through your choice of motions — or actions.
Dr. George W. Crane

The message is clear. Go through the right motions today and you'll soon begin to feel the corresponding emotions. If you choose to smile, you'll feel happier. If you eat right for weight loss, you'll feel thinner. And you'll feel something else just as important, you'll feel in control. You will be the manager of your day. You'd welcome that feeling, wouldn't you?

You may think, "Why should I go around with a false grin on my face if I feel awful? That's dishonest!" Don't kid yourself. What's honest is what you do. It's just as honest to work at being happy as it is to work at being grim. Each is work. Each is your choice. But positive Action will create positive emotions. For example, abstain from overeating and you'll feel happier and lose pounds. That's the whole point, isn't it?

Whenever you make a choice today, ask yourself, "Is this a positive action?" Be in charge. Feel yourself growing more confident, more effective and successful as the pounds drop away revealing an energized you underneath. You'd like that, wouldn't you?

What have you done right today? You learned that motion equals emotion. You see that if your Action is constructive, you will feel good about who you are. Nothing, absolutely nothing, is a bigger challenge.

Today's Action Plan: I will take positive Action. I will be the manager of my emotions today.

The Ninth Action MindStep

...make sure that what you aspire to accomplish is worth
accomplishing, then throw your whole vitality into it
. . . .We must give not only our hands to the doing of it,
but our brains, our enthusiasm,
the best — all — that is in us.

B. C. Forbes

The ninth Action MindStep says: **Take weight loss in steps.** That common-sense idea can get lost in an overweight's natural desire to be instantly thin. We overeaters — often to our detriment — place time limits on our goals; give this or that diet so much time to work its magic, and no more. We tend to live by the calendar, rather than by the goal. Permanent weight loss results from setting one small goal, reaching it, setting the next small goal, and so on. It is a process, a journey. You know that, don't you?

Success is not measured in days, but by accomplishment. In the past you lived by the calendar and were vulnerable to imaginary failures. "After all the time I spent on this diet," you said, "I should have lost more." Such frustration puts you in danger of overeating again.

There is a better way. Set small, attainable weight goals, and live by the goal, not the calendar. Then give it the best that is in you, brains, heart, and hands. Give 100 percent today, won't you?

What have you done right today? You set small, reachable weight-loss goals so you can experience a series of successes. You are now following your own goals, not numbers on a calendar.

Today's Action Plan: I will set weight goals that I can attain, one after the other. I will put no time limits on my success.

Going All the Way

One can go a long way after one is tired.
French Proverb

A successful author once said, "There are mornings when I'm not in a writing mood. In fact, I actually dread facing my typewriter. I procrastinate, rearrange the pens on my desk, stare out the window, even toy with the idea of taking the day off. Finally, I just make a start. To my surprise, these are often my most productive days."

Like that writer, you too need to accomplish, don't you? Sure, it's hard some mornings to face a disciplined day with right-eating, exercise, and attention to developing more comfortable mental attitudes. But from past self-knowledge, you know you must accomplish your goals or you're going to feel far worse.

No one but another overeater knows how you feel when the sun sets on a day lost to overeating. You berate yourself and hate yourself. A day of food indulgence is just not worth the disgust you feel afterwards, is it?

You are stronger now than ever before. When you think you can't face another day of eating right for weight loss, you can. When you think you can't exercise, you can. When you believe you can't change your life, you can. You have what it takes to achieve your goals, don't you? Say YES.

What have you done right today? You were reminded that nothing makes you feel better about yourself than doing what you know you should for your body and your life.

Today's Action Plan: I will go far no matter how tired I am. I will believe I can do what I must.

July 22

The Tenth Action MindStep

Unjust criticism is a disguised compliment. It often means that you have aroused jealousy and envy.

Dale Carnegie

The tenth Action MindStep says: **Reject rejection firmly and totally.** In the past, we've allowed criticism and its implied rejection to almost destroy us. How many times have you overeaten because of a hostile sneer, a sharp word, or an unkind look? How many times?

As overeaters, our former response to criticism was to eat, wasn't it?

Now you are coping with criticism. You are learning to shrug off rejection, firmly and totally. But if you haven't quite handled it yet, try making pearls of rejection.

Oysters handle irritation well. When an irritating little grain of sand works its way inside the shell, the oyster covers it, protecting itself, while forming a beautiful pearl in the process.

When an irritant gets under your skin, make pearls; cover it over with the triumphant, take-charge life you're living. Think of the new harmony between your physical and mental self as a lovely, glowing pearl that no criticism or rejection can ever destroy. Soon you'll have a string of pearls, won't you?

What have you done right today? You refused to allow any destructive criticism or rejection to get under your skin.

Today's Action Plan: I will reject rejection. I will make a pearl out of the criticisms of today.

July 23

Past Remembering

It is not true that suffering ennobles the character;
happiness does that . . . suffering for the most part
makes men petty and vindictive.
                                    W. Somerset Maugham

Dwelling upon our former unhappy overeating life is not wise. But it's worthwhile occasionally to recall those days, to remember overeating as something we certainly don't want to repeat. You do remember, don't you?

Overeating drained you of everything you might have had: health, self-esteem, even enough motivation to try for anything better.

You knew you were sick in some way, but you didn't know how or why. You were too embarrassed to ask for help. You lied to yourself. You denied that you were compulsive about food, blamed your overweight on other problems — lack of money, a family that didn't understand, or friends who didn't care. You felt humiliated in public most of the time.

All this suffering, sad as it is to remember, was the result of overeating. When you stopped overeating, the sick unhappiness left with the pounds. Now you understand that you must get into Action to receive these benefits.

Oh, what great benefits you've received! Health, self-esteem, the desire to achieve, an aliveness. It's worth remembering how you got this far. It's worth almost anything to stay here, isn't it?

What have you done right today? You realized how far you've come and are determined to go further.

Today's Action Plan: I will never go back to the unhappiness of overeating. I will remind myself of the unhappy past, just so each today will be unforgettably good.

The Eleventh Action MindStep

I beg you do not be unchangeable.

Sophocles

Overeaters too often think they are incapable of self-improvement. The eleventh Action MindStep says: **Don't fight inevitable change.** This Action principle urges you to open yourself to hope. You can see hope is the catalyst in our weight-losing formula, can't you?

Perhaps in the past you said, "I failed to lose this weight so many times, I no longer believe it's possible for me." Hold on there! Don't insist on defeat. This kind of hopeless thinking slams the door on new information and new opportunities for change that come along each day.

Change is inevitable. You can't shut it out, so use it. The idea that you can't change your life for the better is to see yourself as the most helpless of creatures, to disown responsibility for whatever happens.

You are capable. Go ahead, experiment with change. Try new exercises. Try new, healthful, body-building foods. Learn to love change. It's the one thing that gives us a chance to choose something better for our lives. Make a good change in your life today, won't you?

What have you done right today? You learned that change is your hope for a thinner-winner future. Rather than being a threat, change is an exciting, ever new friend.

Today's Action Plan: I will not fight inevitable change. I will open myself to everything new, hopeful, and exciting.

July 25

It's Never Ideal

*It's always cold backstage and hot onstage, or some-
body's coughing in the audience, or somebody's beeper
just went off. Or maybe you just played five concerts in
the last five days, and you're tired. It's never ideal, and
that's part of the kick, the fun of performing —
improvising your way out of a hole!*

Eliot Fisk

You may not be a world-renowned guitarist like Eliot
Fisk, but you share his problems. You, too, have to
perform each day even though the circumstances are
never ideal. Can you see that?

Some days are too cold or too hot. Some days people
don't respond to you as you wish they would. Even
though your self-esteem is no longer based on the
approval of others — well, it would be nicer if they paid
you more attention, wouldn't it? And then there are the
days you're just plain tired, cranky, and balky as a
toddler.

Situations are never ideal, but that's part of the
challenge of a take-charge life. What would be the
challenge, or the reward, if it all came easily?

You have both challenge and reward. You have the
fun of performing on your instrument, your body, every
day, no matter what the circumstances. Growing more
physically and mentally fit each day is your way of
making beautiful music, isn't it?

What have you done right today? You see that you
have to move forward positively and perform well, no
matter how trying the circumstances.

**Today's Action Plan: Ideal or not, I will make today
work for me. I will not allow any circumstance to stop
me.**

The Twelfth Action MindStep

Success is the reward for accomplishment.
                                        Harry F. Banks

Play life to win, declares the twelfth Action MindStep. No one suggests that you step over anyone to climb to success. This MindStep merely tells you not to defeat yourself. You'd like a further explanation, wouldn't you?

Overeaters have plenty of energy, but too often it's purely negative energy. We cry, "What's the use? I can't do it!" This book shows you how to convert defeatism into victorious energy, the kind that urges, "Keep going!" "Move ahead!" There it is, the difference between losing and winning.

Don't let wanting to be a winner make you feel guilty. Why should you feel guilty about wanting to look and feel terrific?

Take a really close look at the people around you. Who are the people you admire? Who are the men and women you want to be like? Whether they are successful in weight loss, in business, or elsewhere, they are amazingly alike: winners learn from failure, are self-constructive critics, never blame luck or others, persist no matter what, and experiment with change. Play life to win, won't you?

What have you done right today? You are determined to channel your energy into the winning kind of life you admire in others. That's a wonderful ambition.

Today's Action Plan: I will turn negative into positive energy. I will think like a winner, act like a winner, be a winner.

The Most Powerful Energy You Have

Nothing in the world can take the place of persistence. Talent will not; nothing is more common than unsuccessful men with talent. Genius will not; unrewarded genius is almost a proverb. Education alone will not; the world is full of educated derelicts. Persistence and determination alone are omnipotent.

Calvin Coolidge

Do this one thing. Make your persistence even stronger than your desire. If the race goes to the person who takes one more step than the competition, then winners are people who persist. Your most powerful positive energy is your persistence. You can't buy it, you can't borrow it, you can't inherit it — you must act on it. You can agree with that, can't you?

You already have an achievement-prone personality. That is one of the reasons you are in such mental anguish over your weight.

If you want to be thin for life, you have to act like a winner every day of your life. Take those characteristics you admire in winners, make them yours, and act on them. Say YES to persistence, won't you?

What have you done right today? You believed that persistence, going one step further, is the most important element of your personality. Nurture it and make it grow!

Today's Action Plan: I will be persistent in all that I do. I will believe that I can do far more than I think I can.

When Enough Is Enough

It takes what it takes.
Alcoholics Anonymous saying

Why is it that some people gain ten pounds, hit the panic button, and search for a solution, while others may put on a hundred pounds before the pain propels them into Action? No one knows why people have different levels of pain tolerance. We do know that the same solution works for all overeaters, no matter the size of their problem. It isn't a new magic diet. The permanent solution for overeaters is a new way to see the world and their place in it. Have you ever thought of the MindSteps as a new window to the world?

The negative compulsive personality (many overeaters seem to fall into this category) is marked by passiveness, anxiety, perfectionism, super-sensitivity, and hiding sadness behind a happy-clown exterior. This is the way compulsive people respond emotionally to the world, and in addition, compulsive overeaters buffer these feelings with excess food.

To win your new body, mind, and life you must experience a complete psychic change. Each day you must become more Action-oriented, more confident, more able to learn from mistakes and begin again, more able to reject rejection, and more emotionally honest with yourself and others. Ahh, now you're becoming addicted to this new way of viewing life, aren't you?

What have you done right today? You resolved to make a constructive psychic change, so that you will never have to use excess food to help you face another day.

Today's Action Plan: I will be constructively addicted today. By taking charge of my tendency toward compulsiveness, I can use it to change my life.

Recipe for Success

*Take the obvious, add a cupful of brains, a generous
pinch of imagination, a bucketful of courage and daring,
stir well, and bring to a boil.*

Bernard M. Baruch

Sometimes the obvious — whatever is in plain sight — is
hardest to see. For overweights, it's a set of shiny tools.
Don't ignore all those tools which have proved helpful in
the past. Incorporate them into your successful new plan
for right-eating, exercise, and take-charge attitudes. That
makes good sense, doesn't it?

You may not want to repeat the old diets you tried,
but you can use whichever tools helped you. Keep food-
intake charts, menu and behavior diaries, or exercise
logs. They helped show your progress on paper.

Be ready to reuse old tools and learn new ones too.
After you've lost your excess pounds, overweight will no
longer be an immediate problem. You'll have extra time,
energy, and creative mind-power to spend on other
things. What will you do? Think about it. What have
you always wanted to do but didn't dare think you
could? Plant an expectation that anticipates your
achievement of a thin body, won't you?

What have you done right today? You looked back
and decided to use the tools which worked for you
before. But you're also ready to learn new things for the
happy day when overweight is no longer your most
important problem.

**Today's Action Plan: I will use whatever tools help
me. I will think of the wonderful things ahead.**

Goal Saboteurs

The great pleasure in life is doing what people say you cannot do.

Walter Bagehot

Even the most well-meaning people can unintentionally sabotage our goals. "Don't you think you're getting a little too thin, my dear?" one will ask. We may be many pounds from our natural weights, but because we have changed, others feel threatened. It's important to remember that our own stability would be threatened if someone close to us changed drastically. Therefore, be sure to tell your family and friends that, even though you're changing your weight and your life, they — the persons who are close to you — are more important to you than ever. You can see that they need to be reassured of their place in your life, can't you?

Watch out for the most persistent saboteur of all — you. Compulsive people are often perfectionists, and too often perfectionists think nothing is good enough. Don't try to sabotage yourself by shifting your weight goal as you approach it, making it unattainable. Don't sabotage your weight goal by demeaning it as you come close, so that reaching it is no triumph.

You can't let others, or yourself, sabotage your goal of a thin body, and physical and mental fitness. Be a friend to yourself. The payoff is a marvelously energized way of life. Sounds wonderful, doesn't it? Say YES.

What have you done right today? You saw that others may try to sabotage your weight-loss program, because they feel uncomfortable with your changes. Reassure them and move your own way.

Today's Action Plan: I will not let anyone sabotage my weight goal. And I won't sabotage my own weight goals because "they're not good enough."

Thank Yourself

The search for truth is really a lot of good fun.
                                                Vernon Howard

Say thanks to yourself. Thank yourself for caring enough to give yourself another chance, and for your increased vitality. Thank yourself for the new confidence that got rid of old fears, and for the desire to win that you thought you'd lost. Thank yourself for taking a new course, so you no longer float anchorless from day to day, and for achievable weight goals. Thank yourself for the idea that you can play life to win. It's appropriate to feel grateful to yourself, isn't it?

You have been given another day filled with the promise of achievement. Accept it and the responsibility to keep positive structure in your life. Everything you've achieved so far depends on maintaining mental and physical discipline: eat for weight loss, exercise for health, and practice attitudes of self-respect.

When you do what you know you should do, you are self-trusting, free from the fear that you will overeat. You feel a sense of peace and security.

There is no food sweet enough to tempt you from what you have this day. That's absolutely true, isn't it?

What have you done right today? You thanked the one uniquely wonderful person responsible for your winning life, yourself.

Today's Action Plan: I will remember that I am my best friend. I will not exchange the peace and security of today for any food on earth.

Dream, and It Might Come True

Imagination is more important than knowledge.
Albert Einstein

Imagination is a directed daydream. You allow your mind to play with mental pictures of yourself achieving your wants: a thinner body, contentment, a drive to win. If, as we overweights constantly have been told, we are what we eat, then most certainly we are what we think. You can count on it. Everything you imagine has an incredible power for positive or negative impact. Are you beginning to believe that?

If you use your imagination negatively, you are poisoning your mind against yourself. You tell yourself, "You can't do that." You've been saying that for too long. Please stop hiding fantastic capability behind all those "I can'ts."

If you believe constructively, daydream affirmatively, you're priming yourself for the achievement that will be yours. Positive daydreaming confirms that you'll do whatever good you imagine. Positive imagination can be turned on with practice. Use that same energy to form a positive, affirming image of yourself. Train to be a winner. Put your imagination to work for you. Don't you think it's worth a try?

What have you done right today? You have discovered that positive imagination can be learned and practiced until it is yours. Now you own it.

Today's Action Plan: I will imagine a new life for myself. I will take charge of my imagination, and get rid of the "I can'ts."

August 2

Aliveness

Do not mistake what your life work is; it is your life.
Jo Coudert

When this day is done will you look back and exclaim, "How alive I was then!"? Try to remember days when you felt gloriously alive. What did you do to make yourself feel that way? You'd like to have many such great days, wouldn't you?

Enthusiasm is one way to boost your sense of aliveness. The word "enthusiasm" comes from a Greek word meaning "to be possessed by the god." Think about that. Now, become possessed by enthusiasm. Tell yourself, "This is a wonderful day!" If you act enthusiastic, you can't help but be enthusiastic.

You can measure your aliveness another way. Answer these questions: How much do you want to learn today? How many things do you want to do today? If you are eager to learn, and eager to get into Action, you tingle with aliveness.

If you want more, do more. Isn't it wonderful to discover such a simple solution? You're whipping up enthusiasm right now, aren't you?

What have you done right today? You see that your day rests firmly in your hands, that you can be as alive as you make up your mind to be. You know that you and only you can live your life.

Today's Action Plan: I will look back on this day and say "How alive I was!" I will let the god of enthusiasm come alive in me.

August 3

The Caffeine Consequence

The best way out is always through.
Robert Frost

Sooner or later you'll have to make a conscious health decision about caffeine. Because they use over-the-counter diet pills, as well as drinking diet cola, coffee, and tea which can contain caffeine, people on weight-losing plans seem to consume higher doses of this drug than the average person. You'll know if you're getting too much: insomnia, restlessness, irritability, nervous tremors, and headaches are a few of the symptoms. Bad enough, but there are other caffeine consequences for overeaters. You'd like to know more, wouldn't you?

In small doses, caffeine is a mild stimulant. So if you are a moderate user (two cups of coffee, or one cup and one cola drink per day), you probably don't have much to worry about. But if you overdo (and you *are* prone to overdo, aren't you?), caffeine can produce a chemical brain reaction that is scarcely distinguishable from schizophrenia. That's bad news for overeaters who are trying to channel their thinking into positive mental activities.

It's your choice, whether or not to reduce or omit all forms of caffeine from your diet. It's always your choice. Make a decision that will increase your sense of wellness. Make it today, won't you?

What have you done right today? You checked to see if your symptoms indicate you are getting too much caffeine. You made a conscious decision to get rid of any deterrent to your thinner-winner life.

Today's Action Plan: I will look for real energy in right-eating and exercise. I will get rid of any substance that can keep me from my goals.

August 4

Next Time

You become a champion by fighting one more round.
James J. Corbett

Overweight people are tough taskmasters with themselves. If friends have off days, or even make bad mistakes, you rush to their defense; you reassure them and try to help them be more objective, less self-critical. But if that errant person is you, you probably jump on yourself with both feet. "You big dummy! You never do anything right," you might say. Unfortunately, you do scold yourself that way, don't you?

If, for some reason, your plans for today aren't completed, give yourself a next time. If you set a goal and miss it, give yourself a next time.

Talk back to that negative critic inside you. When it says, "You're whipped, you'll never be thin," answer right back. Say out loud, "That's not true! I can fight one more round." Block out your critical voice by tuning in on your friendly voice.

Your negative voice is the gloomy part of you that expects failure. When it speaks, remember, there is no such thing as total failure — not today, not in a lifetime. Keep slugging one more round and you win the championship of your life. Don't you see that? Of course you do, champ.

What have you done right today? You see that when you don't reach your goal, you must answer the bell for the next round. You deserve another chance, an infinity of chances. Believe.

Today's Action Plan: I will talk back to my negative critic. I will give myself a next time whenever I need it.

August 5

Why You Feel Bad

Every bad feeling you have is the result of your distorted negative thinking.
Dr. David D. Burns

There's an interesting cause-and-effect aspect to bad moods. You probably believed that your depression caused negative thinking. Quite the opposite is true. Negative thinking caused your bad feelings; thoughts cause moods. Did you think it was the other way around?

Some of us had such a negative fix that we didn't even realize it when we were thinking negatively. It was like flying through a storm with a negative automatic pilot system, rarely able to reach the good weather.

If, for a day or so, something good happened to us and we'd burst into the blue, we would say, "That's just a fluke, a mistake. It doesn't count." Then back down we'd dive into the stormy weather, homed-in on our negative thinking radar beam.

Don't make life decisions based on negative self-worth. There's a first-class person in you. Turn off the negative automatic pilot and take control of your own direction. You can take off weight if you program "I'm worth it" thoughts into your flight pattern. Say YES to that, won't you? You've got the right stuff.

What have you done right today? You learned that your destructive thoughts cause your bad feelings and not vice versa. You are determined to steer into the sunshine and stay there.

Today's Action Plan: I will think that I'm a first-class person; therefore I will be a first-class person. I will have nothing but good feelings today.

August 6

Puppets or Puppeteers

Life affords no higher pleasure than that of surmounting difficulties, passing from one step of success to another, forming new wishes and seeing them gratified.
Dr. Samuel Johnson

Have you ever watched a puppet show? Sometimes the dolls are so lifelike that you forget someone is pulling the strings. Then when the show ends, the puppeteer releases control and the puppets collapse to the stage without a life of their own. Have you ever thought of your body as a puppet and your mind as the puppeteer?

You are attached to your puppeteer mind by invisible strings called thoughts. If your thoughts are constructive, your role will be creative; if destructive, you will fall in a heap. You are both puppet and puppeteer. There are both negative and positive strings. Which will you pull?

Each day brings you one step closer to success, to the thinner, energized body and mind you want. Each day the master puppeteer, your positive self, forms new goals and goes after them. Make today's show a celebration of your triumphant life. Do that, won't you?

What have you done right today? You see how inextricably your mind guides your body. You see that your life is a series of thoughts acted out.

Today's Action Plan: I will be a master puppeteer of the good life. I will pull my own strings.

August 7

Doubters Unmasked

If you would have things come your way,
run after them.

Anonymous

If you want success, be a doer, not a doubter. Doubters think nothing will work, therefore, why try? Doubters are belittlers. They ask, "You don't believe that old idea, do you?" Doubters put all their energy and time into bursting other people's bubbles. They never get around to doing anything themselves. They are masters of negative energy. You've known some doubters, haven't you?

Doubters are usually made, not born. They don't want much out of life, don't expect much, and they become very good at negative expectations.

Although doubters appear to be aggressive, they are really very passive and fearful. Don't listen to the doubters. Especially don't listen to your own self-critical doubts.

When you were young you possessed great enthusiasm for trying new things. As a toddler beginning to walk, you took more risks in one hour than most adults take in a year. What's the difference between your infant and adult selves? As an infant, you had curiosity and faith in yourself. You were a doer, not a doubter, and you will be a doer again. How about starting today?

What have you done right today? You are convinced that doubting destroys enthusiasm for living. You are determined to be a doer and to reach the thinner-winner's circle.

Today's Action Plan: I will not listen to doubters. I will have the self-trust and faith that I had as a child.

August 8

Let Go

*A great burden falls away if we let God
run the universe.*

Robert Cummings

There are overeaters who escape the wreckage of their own lives by managing everyone else's. They aren't people who contribute to others' welfare solely out of compassion, but overeaters who find escape in good works. They have time, energy, and advice for everyone else, but their own lives are falling apart. They pretend inner strength while desperately seeking the compliments of others. Even while they take on more and more work, they feel abused by others' dependence. It's a strange process, almost always ending in a destructive food binge. It's true, isn't it?

Are you trying to run everything — others' lives, the whole universe? Scattering all your energy on others as a cover-up for not facing yourself is a losing proposition.

What sad tricks we play on ourselves. What energy we use to smother the mental conflict between what we know and what we do. You're sick and tired of feeling sick and tired, aren't you? Of course, you should help others in need, but concentrate on taking care of your own problems, won't you?

What have you done right today? You learned that if you dissipate all your energy to take charge of others' lives, you are not in charge of your own.

Today's Action Plan: I will put my own house in order, and leave the universe to God. I will concentrate all my energies on setting my own life straight.

Act Smart

*All the world's a stage and all the men and women
merely players . . .*

William Shakespeare

Even if you were never in a play, chances are you have secretly imagined yourself in the spotlight, wowing audiences, getting curtain calls. Isn't that so?

We are all actors. In the morning we put on our costumes (clothes), and get our faces ready (makeup/shave). Then we step out into the world and perform. We smile, gesture, deliver lines. Our audience is made up of our employers, coworkers, family members, and friends.

But actors, even the finest professionals, must have a good script for a good performance. They must study and memorize their lines and deliver them with their best effort.

In your hands you hold award-winning lines, the Twelve Action MindSteps. You know what it takes to win applause from yourself and your audience. Study the lines, memorize them, and then act them out with all your heart. You're ready for your new thin role, aren't you?

What have you done right today? You have decided to start acting the way you want to be. You have discovered the right role and the right lines to make you a winner. Take a bow.

Today's Action Plan: I will walk out on the stage of life and act like a winner. I know I will be a winner because now I have the right lines, the Twelve Action MindSteps.

Relax and Recharge

When your day is largely made up of energetic, concentrated effort, provide for periods of complete relaxation when you can take it easy and recharge your batteries.
Glenville Kleiser

When we rid our days of excess food, we feel more free from tension, stress, and strain than ever before. But because we are compulsive in much that we do, we are in jeopardy of plunging too fast into our new life of physical and mental fitness. If you are living days of highly concentrated effort, you should include daily relaxation. You could use an hour off, couldn't you?

What helps you to relax physically and mentally? Do it today. Do you like to watch two-handkerchief movies on television, or take a walk, or lie on your back in the grass? Do whatever helps you feel free from strain and at ease with your mind and body.

Each day give yourself some time to renew your strength and energy. This will keep your enthusiasm high so you can go back to doing what you want, doing it even better. The few moments you spend unwinding will yield great benefits. Don't you agree?

What have you done right today? You learned to plan for necessary rest, not just sleep at night, but a rest period for your spirit.

Today's Action Plan: I will make time to relax and be at ease with myself. I will refresh myself for what I must accomplish with the rest of the day.

Your Eating Vocabulary

If we change our lives we must first change our attitudes.
The most important thing in our lives is what we are
doing now.

Anonymous

Most people think (and sometimes we overeaters agree)
that overweights consume a wide variety of foods, that
we are gourmets, if you will. But, with few exceptions,
that image is unreal. Most of us have a limited eating
"vocabulary." We eat a small variety of the wrong
things, wrongly prepared foods laden with fat, sugar,
and salt. That's often true, isn't it?

You're not stuck with yesterday's food choices. The
most important thing in your life is what you're eating
today, and today you're changing your eating vocabulary. You've learned to ask for broiled and steamed
food. You say, "No, thank you," to sugar, fat, and salt.

At a recent international Overeaters Anonymous con-
ference in Los Angeles, California, a rumor swept the
hotel that there was fresh broccoli on the dinner menu.
Mouths watered. Lines formed early at the dining room.
It's safe to wager that the hotel had not expected this
group to ooh and ahh over a vegetable as if it were the
most expensive continental pastry.

Eating vocabularies can be changed. You can change
yours. Yesterday's choices don't count, today's do.
You're going to ask for right foods to energize your new
life, aren't you?

What have you done right today? You know that you
can change your eating vocabulary to reflect the real you
that is emerging.

Today's Action Plan: I will drop the words sugar, fat,
and salt from my eating vocabulary. I will eat for a
healthy body.

August 12

Cause and Effect

We are happy because we smile.
William James

Which comes first, the smile, or happiness? According to the law of cause and effect, we should smile after we become happy. Nonsense! We are actually in control of our own happiness because we are in control of our smiles. You have to be convinced of that one, don't you?

Try this: stand in front of a mirror and smile. That's right, just stand there and smile. Keep on doing it, even if you're depressed. Confess now, it's impossible to continue your depression while you're standing there grinning at yourself, isn't it? You can change your attitude by changing your action. The more you smile, the more you feel like smiling.

Add this little rhyme to your smiling act: *stand up tall and straight if you're feeling second rate.* Replace that slouch with height, so you pull up out of yourself. And believe it or not, you'll begin to feel excellent!

You know that if you frown, you feel more like frowning and vice versa. It's really common sense. You become what you do. If you smile and stand tall, you become a happier, more confident person. It's just as simple as that, isn't it? Say YES and smile for yourself.

What have you done right today? You learned that you can't be depressed with a smile on your face. If the smile isn't real at first, it will become real. You won't be able to stop the happiness.

Today's Action Plan: I will smile more. I will stand straight and tall.

August 13

A Label You Can Live With

Worry never robs yesterday of its sorrows; it only saps today of its strength.

A. J. Cronin

Size labels — how they hurt! Labeling may have started in the schoolyard. "Hey, fat stuff!" Later in teen years, "If you'd only take off weight, you could have a date for the dance." Later still, "Sorry about that promotion, but — er, ah — we need a different image." Labels! You're sick of being stereotyped because of your size. You've had enough, haven't you?

Let go of those unhappy memories. Toss them away. They are yesterday's garbage. Today is the day to shop for a different kind of label — a new, proud label you can wear for the rest of your life.

Find your labels: physically strong, mentally positive, emotionally caring. Now gather all the labels of what you are becoming and put your name on them: worthy, achiever, confident, thin, winner. You can think of more, all deserved. Now apply these labels to yourself without hesitation. You will begin to behave in these new ways. There's a big payoff when you affirm these true images. These are labels you can live with for a lifetime, aren't they?

What have you done right today? You no longer worry about old labels. You found labels which fit you today and you wear them with pride.

Today's Action Plan: I will not allow yesterday's labels to sap today of the strength I need. I will wear only my own labels.

Stay-at-home Exercise

I tried a dozen exercise programs — sweat and pain stuff — but I really did best with an at-home program that I made up myself.

Diet club speaker

Exercise doesn't have to be hard work. You can achieve physical fitness with a moderate level of intensity. You don't have to jog to work, run a marathon, or strain on a Nautilus machine. You don't even have to leave your home if you don't want to. Perhaps you've had trouble sticking to a daily program. If so, you'd like to try something that will work for you, wouldn't you?

Try these at-home exercises: jog in place or from room to room, dance by yourself to fast music, bounce on a small trampoline, pedal an exercise bike, skip rope.

As with all exercise, you don't want to pound yourself to a pulp the first few days. Start slowly, then increase your speed, duration, and repetitions as you improve your condition. The idea is to get moving and keep moving. Spend just twenty minutes night and morning every day. This routine will help you lose weight faster and keep it off better. You'll be stronger, your blood pressure and heart rate will decrease, and your disposition will be sunnier.

It's no secret, you want to be healthier and more attractive. Now think of all that energy trapped in your body. Invest some of it in yourself today, won't you? Say YES. Get moving and get thinner.

What have you done right today? You see that you can exercise for fitness and weight loss in your own home. Oops! There goes the last exercise excuse!

Today's Action Plan: I will do one or more of the at-home exercises. I will get moving and keep moving.

Walk to Weight Loss

Can two walk together except they be agreed?
                                                      Amos 3:3

A group of women recently participated in an experiment. All were overweight and, as the researchers put it, resistant to diets. They were asked to do one thing: walk. They had to walk half an hour a day for one year. That's all. No pills, no lectures, no diets. They ate what they wanted. Some actually increased their food intake during the experiment. You can walk for thirty minutes a day, can't you?

What was the payoff after a year? An average weight loss of twenty-two pounds per person! Remember, nothing else was different except the half hour of walking. Their routine was a mile and a half in thirty minutes (that's moving at three miles per hour).

Walking is the easiest exercise to stick to month after month because it's something you do naturally. You don't have to take special instruction; you already know how to walk. Next, how do you fit more walking into your day? That's easy. Try leaving the car at home for short trips, or park a few blocks from your destination and walk.

Best of all, walk with your mate or friend. It's a wonderful way to socialize and share your thoughts while achieving a winner's fitness. Walk today, won't you?

What have you done right today? You learned that you can lose weight and improve fitness doing something you already know how to do.

Today's Action Plan: I will walk today for thirty minutes. I will exercise to be a winner.

Have You Grown?

*The great aim of education is not knowledge
but action.*

Herbert Spencer

Youngsters love to measure themselves against a mark
on the wall to see how much they've grown. We
overeaters also strive to grow. Reaching our goal is
gratifying, of course. But the great accomplishment for
overeaters is not looking back to see how far we've
come, nor looking ahead to see how far we've got to go,
but growth itself. We grow as we learn. However, what
we learn here or elsewhere means nothing unless we use
it. That's right, isn't it?

Action, activity, is the focus of our attention. It's nice
to see that we're more attractive, thinner, more energetic,
and successful. We recognize and love all the good things
coming to us. After a well-deserved pat on the back,
though, we must continue to do the things which got us
this far. We are not people who can just coast. We must
move determinedly to win or we will zoom backwards
almost at the speed of light.

Put your mark on the wall. Congratulate yourself on
your wonderful growth; you are healthier, happier, and
more successful. Continue every day to put into Action
all the things you've learned. You'll do that, won't you?

What have you done right today? You see that how
tall you are isn't as important as maintaining your new
LifeWay. You're determined to continue the Action that
got you this far.

Today's Action Plan: I will grow taller by following
the Twelve Action MindSteps. I will place my next mark
higher on the wall.

A Calming Thing

*He who cannot change the very fabric of his thought will
never be able to change reality.*

Anwar Sadat

Anger is destructive. It may move us to seek revenge.
But overeaters often take revenge on themselves and get
caught in the trap of spite-eating. Look in the mirror.
How many pounds do you owe to anger?

You can handle anger constructively. For example,
anger channeled into a spirit of competition can improve
your performance. This is using a negative emotion to
your advantage. But far too often overeaters lack the
self-confidence required to turn a negative to a positive.
For them, calmness and serenity is a far better response
to anger than eating.

To put yourself into a serene state, try repeating some
calming words — a mantra, a bit of poetry, a prayer.
Many overeaters use the Serenity Prayer: God grant me
the serenity to accept the things I cannot change, to
change the things I can, and the wisdom to know the
difference.

Be willing to try anything to stop spite-eating. Try to
turn anger into a competitive response, or seek the calm,
serene center that is in you. You can see how this would
be far better than angrily overeating, can't you?

What have you done right today? You determined not
to let anger force you into a fit of overeating. You see
that extra pounds on you doesn't solve problems, and
you've become a problem-solver.

**Today's Action Plan: I will not eat out of spite. I will
find the calm core of serenity within me.**

Helping Others Accept Your Change

Those who bring sunshine to the lives of others cannot keep it from themselves.

James M. Barrie

When you begin to change before your family's eyes, it can upset the intricate family balance. You have had a particular place in this system, physically and emotionally. Strange as it seems, other family members, even if they were unhappy with your weight, *expected* you to remain the person you'd always been. For example, perhaps you have been deferential to others because you have felt guilty about your weight. But changing your appearance and showing take-charge behavior can rock the family boat. You can see how this could happen, can't you?

Some families get very upset. Children can feel abandoned when a permissive parent suddenly shows a healthy self-respect. Spouses can long for the return of their non-threatening mates.

Your family needs your help, and you can give it. Praise them. When they compliment you for your weight loss, tell them, "I really rely on your loving support." Reassure your family. Tell them, "I'm happier, and I know we'll all be happier together, now that I'm not overeating." It's wonderful to be able to help yourself and others, isn't it?

What have you done right today? You reinforced your take-charge attitudes by helping others accept them. Your relationships are changing too, for the better.

Today's Action Plan: I will help my family accept my change. I will never return to the pain of overeating to please others.

Friendly Persuasion

The trouble with most people is that they think with
their hopes or fears or wishes rather than
with their minds.

Will Durant

Surveys show that one third of your support, or hindrance, when you lose weight and change attitudes comes from friends and coworkers. When you begin to change, you realize for the first time that you influence everyone around you. That boosts your self-esteem, doesn't it?

You have a place in the life of everyone who knows you. The closer they are, the more your change will affect them. Conversely, the more casual their involvement, the less your change will interfere with them emotionally.

It is human for others to want to be able to count on what they know, to hold onto continuity in their lives. When you lose weight and change the way you view yourself in the world even the most well-meaning friends can feel threatened. They may even say, "I liked you a lot better when you were heavier," or ask, "Aren't you afraid your legs will turn to cellulite?"

Reassure them that what you are doing doesn't affect your friendship with them. Tell them how important these changes are to you. It won't take long for real friends to accept and admire your efforts. If they can't, if they try to sabotage your new life, walk away from them. They aren't friends, are they?

What have you done right today? You concluded that you will help friends accept your change. If they balk because they've lost an eating buddy, you will walk away.

Today's Action Plan: I will continue my new way of viewing the world and my place in it. I will avoid those who cannot accept my new image.

August 20

The Perfectionist

*You will settle for nothing short of a magnificent perfor-
mance in anything you do, so you frequently end up
having to settle for just that — nothing.*
Dr. David M. Burns

Chances are most thin outsiders would find no connec-
tion between our overeating and our perfectionism. After
all, if we really were such perfectionists, we'd lose
weight. But it's not that simple. As compulsive perfectionists we usually fail to focus on a single goal. Our
desire to show the world how truly worthy we are
causes us to overcommit, overwork, and even over-diet,
recklessly spending energy on many diverse goals. You
can see how perfectionism could dissipate energy without
ever getting you to your right-eating goal, can't you?

Perfectionists want everything at once. They find fault
with others who don't live up to high standards and
impose impossible levels of excellence on themselves.
Actually, perfectionists are scared, insecure, competitive
people. They are unable to forgive mistakes, especially
their own.

For the overweight perfectionist who feels inadequate
and scorned, perfectionism is a desire to be above
criticism. There is no such place, and to seek it means we
don't dare take risks, or make changes; we hang onto
old ways with a death grip. That's not what you want
out of life, is it?

What have you done right today? You know now
how destructive these words are: "You can't do anything
right!" You have learned that perfection is a standard,
not a goal. Perfectionism obscures the real process of
winning, which is Action, and change, and Action again.

Today's Action Plan: I will forgive others' mistakes. I
will forgive my own mistakes and be patient with
myself.

August 21

Hurt Feelings

*Almost all negative feelings inflict their damage only as a
result of low self-esteem.*

Author unknown

Marilyn Monroe and Ernest Hemingway, two world-
famous celebrities, killed themselves. No one could
understand why. Apparently they had everything —
money, fame, talent, adoration — everything except a
sense of their own self-worth. They committed the most
profound act of despair and anger. What misery they
must have felt! You know what it is to hurt, don't you?

Feelings don't always reflect reality. And the worse
you feel, the more your thoughts are distorted. When
you think with your feelings, everything seems out of
proportion, exaggerated. Tasks become too hard, too
big. You think they're so important you become overwhelmed.

You can't help feeling hurt now and then, but you can
help how long you feel hurt. When you begin to express
exaggerated feelings you must cancel hurt feelings with
reality checks. Stop the dramatic, vivid language that
you use. You aren't really "ready to die," "devastated,"
or "never able to hold my head up again." You may feel
hurt for the moment, but you're not going to let negative
feelings get you down for long, are you?

What have you done right today? You saw that
feelings and reality don't always match. You separated
the two in your mind.

Today's Action Plan: I will keep my self-esteem high
so that hurt feelings will not inflict damage. I will cancel
hurt feelings by not overeating because of them.

August 22

Zero In on Guilt

Never let yesterday use up too much of today.
                                                    Will Rogers

Everyone in this world has something to feel guilty about. Guilt nags at the conscience and creates the need to cover it up. We overeaters have a special way of hiding guilt: we bury it under piles of food. That's true, isn't it?

Take charge of your guilt by asking yourself: "Am I really to blame?" When you have a low self-esteem quotient, you often take on guilt that is not rightfully yours. Because you see yourelf as wrong and inadequate, you actually assume someone else's guilt, or create guilt where none exists.

Suppose for a minute that you did something wrong and you should feel guilty. Ask yourself a second question, "Will feeling miserable change the situation?" After you make apologies or restitution, there is nothing more you can do but forgive yourself. Continuing to pay and pay, usually by overeating, can't possibly change things. Get on with your life!

Today is too precious to you to spend on impossible guilt. Spend it on the possible, your new life of right-eating, exercise, and positive mental attitudes. Nothing gets rid of yesterday's guilt like living today as you should live it. You can see that, can't you?

What have you done right today? You realize that old guilt can't be hidden under excess food. You plan to live today so that tomorrow will be guilt-free.

Today's Action Plan: If I am to blame for any wrong, I will make amends. Then I will let go of my guilt and get on with a good life.

The Sting

The people who get on in this world are the people who get up and look for the circumstances they want; and, if they can't find them, make them.

George Bernard Shaw

According to the laws of aerodynamics, the bumblebee, because of its heavy body and short wing span, shouldn't be able to fly. But the bumblebee doesn't know about this theory or law and flies anyway. Ideal conditions don't exist for bumblebees, or for people either. We have to fly with what we've got. You'll look at bumblebees in a different way from now on, won't you?

Fly today, from right where you are. If conditions in your life are not ideal for eating right to lose weight, make the conditions right. Success isn't going to come knocking at your door. True, it's right on the other side, but you're going to have to open the door. If it won't open, kick it in!

Does this sound a little overdramatic? Absolutely not. Don't let anything stand in your way. Overeating was in your way, kept you earthbound, stopped you from taking wing, but today you have a new freedom. If, as in the case of the bumblebee, everything points to your inability to fly, fly anyway. Do it, today, won't you? Say YES.

What have you done right today? You learned that even when conditions aren't right for you to take charge of your life, you can do it anyway.

Today's Action Plan: I will make the conditions I need to eat right. I will fly.

Hiding from the Truth

It is never too late to be what you might have been.
George Eliot

When Queen Elizabeth I of England grew old, she ordered all the palace mirrors removed. This didn't make her any younger; it just allowed her to hide her age from herself. We overeaters play mirror tricks; we don't look in them, or we only look from the neck up and ignore our bodies. What a hopeless task, hiding from truth. The truth insistently intrudes, doesn't it?

"I avoided mirrors," a woman at a TOPS convention confessed. "So it was always a terrible shock when I approached a plate glass store window and was forced to stare at myself. I wanted to run and hide from that hateful image."

You've suffered enough. It is monstrous to think of spending your life hiding from your own image. You can still be what you might have been. Don't block your own way; stand aside and let your desire to be thin overwhelm you.

Your greatest achievements are ahead of you. You do know the way; instinctively you understand what is right for your body, what to do with your life. Eat right for weight loss and health, exercise to energize your day, and practice positive can-do attitudes. There, aren't you proud of yourself?

What have you done right today? You quit hiding yourself from yourself. You invited the truth into your life.

Today's Action Plan: I will not be a barrier to success. I will be what I might have been.

Walk On

True enjoyment comes from activity of the mind and exercise of the body; the two are united.
Alexander Humboldt

Try to become more aware of your thoughts about exercise. Are they real or distorted? Do you think, "I'd look foolish striding around the neighborhood going nowhere"? If you think that way, correct yourself like this: "Nobody cares what I do, and if they do, so what? I want to walk for exercise, and I'm going to do it no matter what." See how you can correct distorted thinking?

Walk for pleasure and for weight-loss. If you're shy, walk before there's a crowd on the street. You will be doing yourself a favor.

Starting early has another advantage. Walking before breakfast (after a twelve to fourteen hour overnight fast) seems to create *faster weight loss.* It may be that walking with an empty stomach makes the body dip into its calorie reserves. One group of women who walked thirty minutes before breakfast, in addition to their evening walk, lost an astounding 42 percent more than a group that walked only in the evening.

Now you're thinking clearly about your right to exercise whenever you want. Be an early bird, won't you?

What have you done right today? You confronted distorted thinking that tells you everyone is watching what you do. You've decided to walk early, walk briskly, and enjoy it.

Today's Action Plan: I will walk for exercise. I will get rid of distorted thinking about exercise, and do it.

Independence

*Let fortune do her worst, whatever she makes us lose, as
long as she never makes us lose our honesty
and our independence.*

Alexander Pope

According to the dictionary, independence means "self-maintenance or self-government." This conjures visions of hardy individualism. But in a sense, the word independence has more in common with self-discipline. Does that alliance surprise you?

Being truly independent means increasing your personal options, not necessarily with the world, but with yourself. An independent, self-maintaining, self-governing person chooses to control his or her thinking, feeling, and Action.

Independence doesn't mean going it alone, or isolating yourself from others. Instead, the more you think and act for yourself, the closer you can be to others because there is a healthy equality.

Each day you don't overeat is a day when you are more of an independent, self-governing person. You are probably finding that increasing your independence from overeating motivates you to make other wise choices. Making wise choices brings you contentment and happiness. Are you happy today? Why not stay that way?

What have you done right today? You see that to be independent is to be self-governing, which gives you the widest possible range of choices in your day.

Today's Action Plan: I will grow toward independence by practicing self-discipline. I will choose to be happy.

The One Attitude that Is You

Seek out that particular mental attitude which makes
you feel most deeply and vitally alive, along with which
comes the inner voice which says, "This is the real me,"
and when you have found that attitude, follow it.

William James

One attitude which is central to your existence says, "I can live today without overeating." That attitude is one that you can follow for your lifetime. Believe this. Belief is a powerful affirmation, confirmed by your Action every day. Instinctively you know this, don't you?

While you were overeating you asked yourself the wrong question: "Do I want to eat this?" Now that you are not overeating, you ask the right questions: "Do I want these excess pounds?" "Do I want to feel miserable?" "Do I want this kind of future?"

These right questions are part of reality thinking. It's what alcoholics call "looking through the bottom of the bottle," which means you are looking past the supposed pleasure of the next bite to the consequences of overeating *before* you eat.

Ask the right questions. Deal with reality. Now you have made yourself available for success by removing the love of excess food from your life. This is the real you, isn't it?

What have you done right today? You identified the attitude that is really you and confirmed it by Action.

Today's Action Plan: I will "look through the bottom of my plate." I will ask myself the right questions when tempted to overeat.

August 28

The Overeater's Personality

Each of us needs time for mental self-renewal.
                                    Whitt N. Schultz

Seven personality traits have been identified with overeaters by the international organization Overeaters Anonymous. How many apply to you?

1. Overeaters have a *low frustration tolerance.* (Every frustration must give way to immediate satisfaction, usually food.)
2. Overeaters are *grandiose.* (They talk and act like bigshots to cover their low self-esteem.)
3. Overeaters are *isolated.* (They are insecure loners.)
4. Overeaters are *over-sensitive.*
5. Overeaters are *impulsive.* (They are intense sprinters, not marathoners.)
6. Overeaters are *defiant.*
7. Overeaters are *dependent.* (They are not only dependent on food, but they lean on others emotionally.)

Think about these overeater traits. If you see yourself in any of them, make positive changes. Self-confidence replaces grandiosity; caring for others replaces isolation; developing a sense of self-worth replaces over-sensitivity; step-by-step goals replace impulsiveness; firmly rejecting rejection replaces pugnacious defiance; take-charge attitudes replace dependence. The Twelve MindSteps give you a positive new profile to work toward. Make today an emotional success, won't you?

What have you done right today? You know that you are what you do, so to change a negative trait, replace it with a positive one.

Today's Action Plan: I will make positive personality changes. I will make today an emotional success.

What You Are

Look to this day, for it is life, the very life of life.
                                                    Sanskrit Proverb

You're a fighter. You never give up. You hold proof in your hands, this book. Quitters don't read self-help material. Winners do. Applause, applause! Go ahead, accept this accolade, won't you?

You're tougher than you know. Because we overeaters are sensitive to the hurts we've felt, we convince ourselves and others that we should be treated carefully. You've been hurt, yes, even cried, but you're not fragile.

"Tough in a crisis." Think of yourself that way. Expect to be strong when the chips are down. If you treat yourself as the person you want to be, you'll become that person.

Seeing adversity as a challenge brought you to this day, a day of choices. You can make it anything you want with your positive thoughts and acts. Just as negative attracts negative, positive attracts positive.

Use your achieving attitudes in each of today's 1,440 minutes, strengthened by your survivor's instincts. Start with your desire, then do the right physical and mental things that will propel you to success. Your Action today will turn desire into reality.

What have you done right today? You realize now that you can handle adversity and come up fighting.

Today's Action Plan: I will never quit. I will use every minute of this day to propel myself toward success.

How You Think of Yourself

Keep in the sunlight.
Benjamin Franklin

Don't think of yourself as only an overweight person. You are so much more than a weight on the scale. Don't let your weight rule your self-esteem. If you haven't shed the weight you wanted to in the time you've allotted, don't make yourself miserable. Have you played that no-win game?

When our script doesn't play the way we write it, we overeaters suffer self-blame and self-humiliation in the belief that we're always wrong. What nonsense!

Stop thinking, talking, and acting depression. Look inside to find your positive self and believe that you are far stronger than your fears.

Stay in the emotional sunlight, affirm yourself to yourself. Focus your emotional energy on your value. Think, "I'm doing something great!" and "I don't have a single doubt in myself."

Set the scene: you know where you're going, you know where to begin. Now move forward and don't quit! That's your script for today. Give a great performance, won't you?

What have you done right today? You recognized that you are not defined by your weight and your self-esteem isn't ruled by your scale. You vowed to write a positive script and then give an award-winning performance. Take a bow!

Today's Action Plan: I will bask in the emotional sunlight of self-worth. I will look deep inside and find strengths I didn't know I had.

Give Yourself Recreation

*People who cannot find time for recreation are obliged
sooner or later to find time for illness.*
John Wannamaker

Recreation is essential to emotional health. It recreates
energy, quickens motivation, increases mental fitness,
brings pleasure, and supplies fond memories. You see
that recreation is more than just entertainment or a way
to fill time, don't you?

Overeating is not a pleasure. It doesn't leave fond
memories, does it? Can you call that uncomfortable,
stuffed feeling, that disappointment in ourselves, that
anguish over weight gain healthy, motivating, energizing, or pleasurable? No!

Learn to laugh again, love yourself again, be comfortable in your own company. It doesn't matter what you
do for recreation, alone or with others, at home or half a
continent away. People who can laugh, love, and enjoy
themselves develop deep confidence and faith in themselves.

Banish distrust and discouragement today. Give yourself the recreating pleasure of abstaining from excess
food. You'll do that, won't you?

What have you done right today? You learned about
the pleasurable benefits of recreation. You became a
person who laughs and loves and can find joy alone or
with others.

**Today's Action Plan: I will give myself pleasure
through recreation — without excess food. I will seek
recreation because it is essential to my health.**

Your Basic Needs and How to Get Them

*Without food, I will die; without food control,
I won't live.*
Overeaters Anonymous member

To find contentment, we need more than the basic life-sustainers: air, food, water, and shelter. Most essential to our happiness are three other basic human needs: to be loved, to be productive, and to be self-valuing. That's quite an assortment, isn't it?

Because these needs are basic to your sense of personal worth, inner pressure compels you to fulfill them. But when overeating is dictator, there is terrible conflict. Food-abuse strikes at almost every basic need! Think about that. When we overeat, we destroy self-worth, productivity, and our ability to love and believe we are loved. We damage our sense of productive creativity because we stunt personal growth.

When you stop overeating, you create a climate in which growth and change can flourish. When you replace negative eating habits with positive ones, you do a natural thing — you fulfill your basic, human needs. When you eat right, exercise, and embrace positive mental attitudes, you feel more comfortable with yourself. Isn't that fulfilling?

What have you done right today? You saw that food-abuse destroys your sense of comfort by denying you your basic human needs. How powerful right-eating can be!

Today's Action Plan: I will not abuse food. I will fulfill my basic human needs and grow more comfortable with myself.

September 2

A Quick Fix for Anxiety

I keep the telephone of my mind open to peace, harmony, health, love and abundance. Then, whenever doubt, anxiety or fear try to call me, they keep getting a busy signal — and they'll soon forget my number.

Edith Armstrong

When you're in conflict with basic needs — sustenance, safety, love, self-esteem, and creativity — anxiety results. And anxiety produces discomfort, helplessness, tension — even panic. You recognize these feelings, don't you?

Overeating is an attempt to escape from anxiety. But like alcohol, drugs, or gambling, food has only a momentary anesthetic effect. You have to keep eating to control the pain of conflict, using larger quantities of food, isolating yourself further from reality.

When your needs conflict, don't press the food panic button. There's a better way, called deliberate relaxation. Sit in a quiet room. Tense all your muscles at once: clench your fists, press your head back against your chair, squeeze your eyes, clamp your teeth, lift your legs to tighten your stomach muscles. Now take a deep breath, hold for a five count, then let everything relax, go limp, and stay limp for several minutes. Concentrate on total relaxation so you'll remember how it feels. This exercise is guaranteed to create a more pleasant memory than a food binge. Don't you think so? Say YES.

What have you done right today? By practicing real physical relaxation instead of overeating, you have done exactly what is right for you.

Today's Action Plan: I will not turn to food as a drug for anxiety relief. Instead I will practice relaxation.

September 3

Be a Food Boss

The smallest action is better than the largest plan.
John Graves

Be assertive with food. Don't be bossed by a bar of candy, bamboozled by a bun, or berated by a butter pat. Even though we overeaters try to laugh about succumbing to temptation ("the devil made me do it!"), when food controls us, it's no joke. No one knows that better than you, isn't that so?

It's time for you to be the food boss. Be assertive. Talk back! When a high-calorie dessert calls to you from the refrigerator, when you hear the sweet tempter's siren song as you pass the baker's case, quietly and firmly tell them no. We overeaters have given food power that we must take back. You can do it.

Be assertive when you eat out. Once you have finished eating what is right for you, don't allow anyone — waiter or hostess — to browbeat you into eating more. Politely but firmly decline to clean up the dish.

Success is a habit, in this case the habit of saying no. Don't let food or other people control your life. Be the boss, won't you?

What have you done right today? You found that being in control of the food you eat gives you a wonderful sense of well-being. You don't feel helpless, but full of take-charge strength.

Today's Action Plan: I will firmly refuse any food that is not on my right-eating plan. I will be the boss.

246

Take Charge of Fat in Your Food

*The moment a question comes to your mind, see
yourself mentally taking hold of it and disposing of it. In
that moment is your choice made. Thus you learn to
take the path to the right. Thus you learn to become the
decider and not the vacillator.
Thus you build character.*

H. Van Anderson

Each day you are making decisions in your life. You
have truly become the driver and not just the passenger.
You are creating your own winning future. You feel
good about being in charge, don't you?

You are already doing something about the fat on
your body. Today, make a decision about the amount of
fat you allow into your body. It's important to confront
the fat content in your food. Increasing scientific evidence links fat in food with heart disease and cancer, and
some research shows it may be more of a problem than
sugar for the overweight.

In a recent experiment, sugar intake accounted for
fewer pounds of extra weight than fats in our food. In
the same experiment, overweight people were shown to
like fatty foods. They preferred cream to milk and liked
heavy cream laced with safflower oil best of all.

The payoff in reducing your consumption of fat is
accelerated weight loss, better health, and probably
longer life. Make your decision for the good life, won't
you?

What have you done right today? You became the
driver, making important fat-reducing decisions about
your health and body. What a great day this is!

Today's Action Plan: I will limit my fat consumption.
I will decide that I'm in charge of my body and my life.

Cope-ability

*Rule No. 1 is, don't sweat the small stuff. Rule No. 2 is,
it's all small stuff.*

Robert Eliot

Anxiety. That's a fancy word for emotional pain — pain
that can be very real, as every overweight knows. How
many times have you said "I just can't stand it anymore!" But you can't avoid painful experiences; everyday
life is full of them, and living fat in today's world is often
less than fun. But overeating hasn't been a good barri-
cade between you and emotional pain in the past, has it?
Overeating just created its own pain. That's true, isn't it?

Overeating works like iodine on a cut — it makes the
hurt worse. So what should you do? Be realistic, for one
thing. Realize that situations and people will upset you
— everything from a stuck drawer to a traffic jam will
upset you. Don't rush to use food as a buffer. Decide to
concentrate on "yes" things that will turn opportunities
into reality. Don't say it won't work until you've tried it.
It's worth a try, isn't it?

What have you done right today? You have learned to
turn anxious moments into assets, failures into successes,
defeats into victories. How? Any day you live without
the emotional buffer of excess food, crown yourself
winner of the day.

Today's Action Plan: I will remember that most of the
problems that prompt me to eat are small stuff. I will
believe that there is no limit to what I can do.

Negative I-grams

Obstacles are those frightful things you see when you take your eyes off the goal.

Hannah More

Are you so enthusiastic about your LifeWay that you won't settle for anything less? If you aren't, check your "I-grams." These are the "I" instructions which form your self-image. When you telegraph negative messages to yourself, such as "I'm no good," "I'm so stupid," or "I'm a fat slob," you make those messages your goal. You can see that, can't you?

Don't make life-decisions based on negative thinking. If you thought, "I feel like a second-class person; therefore I *am* a second-class person," you fooled yourself, tragically.

Be aware of how often you sabotage yourself with "I can't" thoughts. Know how often you feel sad, discouraged, guilty, and disappointed. That's so punishing, and so wrong.

You know it's against the law to mislabel a product. Furthermore, it's just plain bad business to downgrade a good product. So package yourself right. Put a cheerful, positive label on yourself. By sending positive "I-grams" to your self-image, you are merely obeying truth-in-packaging laws. Start right now to think, "I am wonderful," or "I have what it takes to succeed." You'll do that, won't you? Say YES.

What have you done right today? You based life-decisions on positive "I-grams."

Today's Action Plan: I will give myself positive labels. I will keep my eye on my goal, a life without excess food.

September 7

The Convincing Self-critic

There are some people who are very resourceful at being remorseful.

Ogden Nash

"I am worthwhile." Do you cringe, unconvinced, from that truth? Believe it. The quality of your life begins with that belief. Too often we overeaters are so angry with ourselves that we convince others of our lack of worth. With vivid, colorful, ingenious language we persuade family, friends, even professional counselors, that we are rotten people and deserve maximum unhappiness. We fight any tiny sense that we have value. Are you a convincing self-critic?

Even accomplished self-haters can't avoid occasional positive experiences. But what do they do when something wonderful happens? They disqualify it as a fluke. It doesn't count because they don't deserve it. Their negative thinking is ingrained, so they hang on to it with all their strength. It's their way of saying, "I'm so bad inside; if you really knew me, you'd agree that I don't deserve anything good."

Stop being a convincing self-critic. Don't be so fierce with yourself. Refuse to persecute yourself. If you make a mistake today, think, "I'm only human, and the whole of me is not ruined." Give yourself a little peace, won't you? Then go on from here.

What have you done right today? You confronted your convincing self-critic with a demand to stop this persecution. You learned that you deserve a little human kindness — from yourself.

Today's Action Plan: I will not disqualify positive experiences. I deserve the chance to succeed today.

September 8

How to Fight Your Inner Critic

*The world has a way of giving what is demanded of it
. . . .If you look for failure, you will get it . . . .Lack of
faith in yourself, in what life will do for you, cuts you
off from the good things of the world. Expect victory
and you make victory.*

Preston Bradley

Overeaters who make mistakes don't know when to stop
blaming themselves. Their busy inner critics begin to
drum out their negative messages: "Dummy, dummy,
dunce. You've failed again. Might as well accept it —
you deserve to be fat!" Letting your inner critic get the
upper hand can lead to more overeating and more self-
criticism. You'd like to learn how to silence your inner
critic, wouldn't you?

Try this when you've made a mistake and you can't
stop whipping yourself about it. Set a definite time to be
angry about it (five minutes on a timer will do nicely).
Stand in front of a mirror and shout all the things your
nasty inner critic has been thinking. Moan, cry, hit the
wall. When the time is up, stop. The incident is ended.

Funny thing — you won't want to blame yourself
anymore. Long before the end of your five-minute
purge, you'll be tired of it. You'll realize you don't really
believe the rotten things your inner critic was saying.
You're in charge of everything, even your own self-put-
downs, aren't you?

What have you done right today? You want to banish
your self-critic so much, you decided to try your own
scream therapy. Congratulations, for sending an eviction
notice to that noisy, no-good, critical drummer!

**Today's Action Plan: I will defeat my inner critic. I
will take any step to gain victory over overeating.**

Do You Have a Talent for Happiness?

*[Happiness is the] agreement of a person's inner life with
the reality of his outer experience.*
                                                    William James

This quote means that happiness is achieved by express-
ing your inner values through doing what you feel you
must do. If this sounds familiar, it should. This book is a
365-day tribute to this principle. One way to create
happiness is to achieve harmony between what we want
(to stop overeating) and what we actually do (right-
eating, exercise, and attitude). When we create harmony
between our ideals and our actions, we are in James'
"happy agreement." Put this way, happiness sounds
quite simple, doesn't it?

Some people have a special talent for achieving happiness. They work constantly for what they want and
accept nothing less. They enjoy the excitement of challenge. They are confident in their values, and believe
their lives have meaning and direction. They are self-
directed, without conflict, and at peace.

You too are good at happiness. When you get rid of
the need for excess food, you will enjoy life regardless of
setbacks. You'll get more out of everything you do
today. The circumstances are just right for a LifeWay
that features right-eating, body exercise, and winning
attitudes.

To the extent that you take charge of your life, you
are open to happiness. Open the door all the way, won't
you?

What have you done right today? You put your ideals
and actions in agreement by right-eating. You know it is
a beginning which makes future happiness possible.

Today's Action Plan: I will develop my talent for
happiness. I will get the most out of today by controlling
my desire for excess food.

That's Not the Way It Feels

Although words exist for the most part for the transmission of ideas, there are some which produce . . . violent disturbance in our feelings . . .
Albert Einstein

More than once you've heard a person say: "She doesn't mind being fat. Why, she laughs and makes jokes about it herself." Did you ever want to tell that person, "That's not the way it feels; she laughs to cover up the hurt"?

It hurts to feel like an outsider, and we laugh to show it doesn't matter. It hurts to be excluded from the party, and we pretend we're too busy to go anyway. It hurts not to have a sweetheart, so we fabricate one who always happens to be out of town. We may rationalize, or may joke and laugh about being overweight (we do it first, so no one else will) but that's not the way we really feel. No one should live that way.

Today hurtful words cannot harm you. You are eating to live, instead of living to eat. Isn't it wonderful that happiness is not based on what you hear about yourself, but what you know about yourself?

Happiness — real fun and laughter — is a natural state for your healthy mind. You can make it a permanent state of mind by following your three-part plan: right-eating, energizing your body with exercise, and concentrating on the Action MindSteps.

Today is glorious. Enjoy it. Think of this day as the day you've always looked forward to. You feel great! That's the way you should feel, isn't it?

What have you done right today? You didn't have to laugh to cover hurt. You loved the real laughter that your new LifeWay made possible.

Today's Action Plan: I will not be disturbed by others' words. I will feel great today, making happiness my natural state of mind.

Help Yourself to a Bigger Portion of Life

Life is either daring adventure or nothing.
Helen Keller

You can change your self-image. Yes, you can. Self-image is composed of the accumulated impressions of your life, and these can be changed by gathering new and different impressions. We gather impressions from others and from our own observations. It is important to have the best self-image we can create because our self-image directs the way we act. You believe that, don't you?

People who successfully recreate their self-image share important personality traits. They have positive attitudes, are receptive to life changes, and feel personally responsible for their own health. These people can also recreate themselves physically because they are in tune with their bodies. They have body-awareness because they focus their attention on the physical changes they want to make.

Winners can create and hold a positive self-image and sense how they will feel after accomplishing their goal. They can "taste success."

You are eating for health and happiness, piling up positive impressions for your new self-image. Are you ready to be transformed into a winner? Say YES.

What have you done right today? You gathered new, positive, responsible, well-focused, successful impressions.

Today's Action Plan: I will recreate myself with a positive self-image. I will gather winning impressions.

Toward Personal Growth

I'm a normal, narcissistic, egotistical person with all sorts of vanities. Underneath my mirror there's a little sign that says, "This person is not to be taken too seriously."

Dr. Lawrence Mintz

Being overweight in a thin-is-in culture is no laughing matter. But it doesn't do any harm if, every now and then, you take yourself and your problem just a little less seriously. You could stand a little more sunlight, couldn't you?

There's much to be said for a brighter outlook. If you can laugh at the little obstacles, you can rebound faster and feel less frustration. Laughter is great for taking the steam out of anger, allowing your self-worth to rise.

Work on your weight problem, but see the humor around you at the same time. With a sense of humor you'll look at your problems differently, not get so beaten down, be able to bounce back.

Being able to see humor in a situation is quite different from making yourself the butt of "fat jokes." Self-put-downs only increase tension, whereas humor releases tension. You've got the idea. Now have fun. You deserve it, don't you?

What have you done right today? You decided to relax and laugh a little. You put more light moments into your day.

Today's Action Plan: I will see the humor in life's situations. I will not take myself so seriously.

September 13

Are You Always Wrong?

To the extent that a person fails to attain self-esteem, the consequence is a feeling of anxiety, insecurity, self-doubt, the sense of being unfit for reality, inadequate to existence.

Nathaniel Branden

You program yourself. What you program into your mind, you'll get out. In data processing, there's a well-known warning against careless programming: Garbage in, garbage out. What's true of a computer is true of your mind. Believe that, won't you?

The lowest form of mental garbage is: "Whatever I am, is wrong." With that program you can't possibly believe anyone could like or accept you. With that input, you can go one of two ways: become a doormat, begging people to step on you, or become so aggressive (proving how rotten you really are) that your behavior makes you an outcast. Either way you are apt to overeat.

Here's your new Action MindStep program titled: "Whatever I am, is right." With your new program loaded into your memory bank, you have a solid belief in your own worth. Anxiety is replaced with confidence, a sense of unreality is replaced with the reality of your right-eating plan, and you are prepared to play life to win. You see how it works, don't you? Positive in, positive out. That's much better, isn't it?

What have you done right today? You got rid of mind-garbage by reprogramming your mental computer with MindStep attitudes.

Today's Action Plan: I will think, "Whatever I am, is right." I will put into my mind what I want to get out.

September 14

Do What You Can — but Do It!

Half of today is better than all tomorrow.
                                                            La Fontaine

Sometimes overeaters think it's impossible to commit themselves in the morning to a full day of right-eating for weight control. If your day stretches out in front of you interminably and you can't make a full commitment, don't wait until tomorrow to take Action. Promise yourself you'll eat right for half a day. Anyone can manage a half-day, right?

Now that you've committed yourself to a half-day's right-eating, you've given yourself extra time, the time you used to spend eating. Use it. Remember that your ability to think is the key to open your life. Your power to think can create new ways for you to live.

Every day, even every half-day, your powerful thoughts create a winning aura around you. These splendid hours that you have excess food out of the way will brighten your whole environment. Don't dwell on your anxiety. Don't fix your attention on depressing conditions. Not once.

You have the power to think, to create, to plan. Use it to tell yourself the truth: what you want is possible. Train yourself to think of possibilities, and when your half-day is past, you won't want to stop. You want to go on, don't you?

What have you done right today? You were willing to give yourself a half-day. You knew that a half of today is more important than all of tomorrow.

Today's Action Plan: I will use my time to create a mental environment that will help me stay free of overeating. I will do it because I have the power to control my life.

September 15

Do You Have Too Many Choices?

*There are no circumstances, however unfortunate, that
clever people do not extract some advantage from.*
                                        La Rochefoucauld

Someone once quipped that if problems are opportunities, there sure are a lot of opportunities around. Maybe
too many for overeaters making a choice about weight-
losing methods. Sometimes we have a problem because
there are so many alternatives. We have to decide
between diet clubs, self-help therapy groups, spas,
salons, hypnotism, clinics, books, TV diet gurus, our
family doctors, powders, pills, shots — and on and on in
a bewildering array of options. It's tough to make a
decision, isn't it?

Here's a formula to help you decide. Ask yourself:
        What do I want?
        What must I do to get it?
        Where do I go?
        When should I start?
You'll eliminate all but a few possibilities. Then give
these, one at a time, a chance to work for you. But don't
let indecision continue for long. Indecision inevitably
leads to overeating.

Today you are in focus, functioning at a winning
level. Your mind is aware, clear, and set on a goal. That
makes decisions possible, doesn't it?

What have you done right today? You have used the
principle of Action to help you make a choice. When
you have a problem, you find a way to work it out,
don't you?

**Today's Action Plan: I will make decisions as quickly
and intelligently as possible. I will focus on winning my
goal of mastery over food.**

September 16

Winning Dreams

Dream lofty dreams, and as you dream, so shall you become. Your vision is the promise of what you shall at last unveil.

John Ruskin

It happened like this. You picked up this book. You began to read a page, anywhere. You read it again and made a decision to start each day with a reading, giving two minutes of your time to yourself. No harm in that, was there?

Before you realized it, you were hooked. You began applying the Twelve Action MindSteps, and you found your view of yourself and your life changing. You plunged into a new LifeWay of right-eating, exercise, and mental fitness.

It's true! This is no dream. Look at yourself. You are losing weight, you feel more attractive and healthier, and your self-esteem has never been higher. This amazing success has expanded into other phases of your life. You win the game, land the job, become more loving and lovable. You, not food, play the leading role in your life. The world is yours!

Is it right to dream such dreams? You bet it is! They inspire you to go for the sweepstakes, the grand prize.

Now go beyond dreams. Blend reverie with Action. You can do it, can't you? You know you can.

What have you done right today? You allowed yourself to dream wonderful dreams. You are ready to move beyond dreams to winning success and a new body.

Today's Action Plan: I will dream of what I want to be. I will make these dreams reality with my Action program.

September 17

Take Responsibility

*Every person is responsible for all the good within the
scope of his or her abilities . . .*
Gail Hamilton

Who are the "they" that we blame? Who are the ones
responsible for our bad feelings, intense anxiety, and
even depression? Overeaters who avoid self-responsibility only magnify their problems. They approach life as if
all events were entirely beyond their control. They feel
manipulated at the hands of "they." Don't you agree?

Take responsibility for your feelings, thoughts, and
actions. If you know you need a change in your life,
take responsibility for making that change. This makes
more sense than living in fear of "they."

You can't always control what happens outside you,
but you can control what happens inside you.

Take charge of your emotional life and build emotional strength. Know your worth. Accomplish your goals.
Stand your ground. Initiate Action. Plan and use your
own time. Bounce back with new energy after confronting a problem.

Handle today's feelings first. Don't swallow them or
you'll surely overeat later. Today express your feelings
responsibly. That's vital! It will make pounds and
pounds of difference. That's true, isn't it?

What have you done right today? You saw that
making "them" responsible for your feelings is self-
destructive. You took charge of today's feelings so there
would be no need to overeat.

**Today's Action Plan: I will control what happens
inside me. I will express my feelings responsibly so that I
will not overeat.**

September 18

A Friend in Need

*We readily welcome to our group of friends that one
who talks with the voice of experience and common
sense. We know that we are safe in his hands. He is not
going to get us into trouble. Rather he is going to point
out the pitfalls and mistakes that experience has taught
him to avoid.*

George Matthew Adams

Do you think being strong means going it alone? Absolutely not! In times of high stress, when you are in danger of overeating, talk to someone who is important to you. Don't turn to food; it's not your friend. Turn to a real friend, a relative, a minister, your teacher, your Twelve-Step group sponsor. You would consider doing this, wouldn't you?

To paraphrase the poet, overeaters cannot be islands unto themselves. We must be willing to seek and accept help when we need it.

There are many benefits. Often you receive feedback from another's experience to help you work out a solution. Even more often, you hear yourself working out your own solution. There's another benefit in asking that special person for help. You feel cared for. That's not too hard to take, is it?

Ask for all the help you need. Then take it, act on it, and make necessary changes in your life. Now you're behaving just like top winners. Isn't this better than being alone?

What have you done right today? You learned you don't have to be an island. You see that it is so much better to turn to a helpful friend than to your food enemy.

**Today's Action Plan: I will discuss stressful events
with someone important to me. I will not eat from
stress.**

Excuses, Excuses, Excuses

*The trick is not how much pain you feel. Life is full of
excuses to feel pain, excuses not to live . . .*
                                            Erica Jong

Overeaters feel pain — the pain of living in a world that
sometimes despises us, discriminates against us, and,
worst of all, laughs at us. Oh, there are plenty of times
for us to feel righteous self-pity. We must resist them all.
Self-pity is an admission that we feel inadequate, helpless, and lonely. Don't you agree?

If you allow today's chances to slip by because you
remember past pain, you are indulging in self-pity and
you are encouraging contentment to fly out the window.
Now is the time to reject rejection, especially your own
rejection of yourself.

Self-pity is a phantom pain, like the pain an amputee
feels in a limb that is no longer there, a remembered pain
that stops us from facing today. It becomes an excuse
not to try.

Burn the past; learn from it and let it go. Don't drag
yesterday's hurts into the future where you can stub
your ego on them. Drop old pain like a bad habit by
understanding how destructive it is. Understanding, not
awareness, is the starting point. Understanding puts you
in charge of your pain, so you can choose to let it go.
Remember?

What have you done right today? You have learned
that self-pity is really self-induced helplessness. Remembered pain can be an excuse not to live today to its
fullest. Get rid of all self-pity.

Today's Action Plan: I will not be diverted by yesterday's pain. I will take charge of any desire to feel sorry
for myself.

September 20

Heart And Soul

Strong convictions precede great actions.
                                                J. F. Clarke

Victory in sports, to some extent, is achieved through the athlete's natural talent and good luck. That is, winning a championship takes more than raw talent and the random bounce of a ball. Titles require heart-and-soul commitment, and the players who have it are rare. In the weeding-out process of competition, players with this special quality emerge again and again as champions. You'd like to know what special quality they have, wouldn't you?

Heart-and-soul commitment is a strength and fiber of spirit. It is something inside you that makes you dig down to discover your true self and act on it.

In your daily struggle for a thinner-winner LifeWay, you have barely touched your innate ability. Do you want to become a champion? Of course you do, with all your heart and soul!

World titles are won with your kind of winner's attitude. They are won by fighters like you who prepare both mentally and physically to win at the game of life, who dig down deep for that something extra when they need it. Believe there's a champion in you, won't you?

What have you done right today? You decided to win the gold medal of life. You are ready to dig deep for that champion spirit to free yourself from overeating.

Today's Action Plan: I will be a MindStep superstar. I will work with all my heart and soul to uncover the winner within me.

You Are Only Responsible for Your Own Feelings

Mama may have, Papa may have, but God bless the child who's got his own.

Billie Holiday

Beware people who try to manipulate you with negative criticism. If what they say is constructive and based on their own successful experience, you can respect and learn from it. But if the criticism is merely an attempt to make you conform to others' ideas, reject it. A recovering overeater must believe this, don't you think?

Sometimes our rejection of their ideas makes others say, "I always give you my best, and you don't appreciate it," or "You make me feel bad when you don't do what I ask."

Don't accept responsibility for anyone else's feelings *if* there is no fault in your behavior. If people try to tell you that what you do makes them unhappy, tell them in a sensitive, but firm way that their feelings are their responsibility.

Some of the negative feedback you get from others may be a disguised request for you to change back to the way you were, or to the way they want you to be. By pleasantly reminding them that they are in charge of their feelings, you put the responsibility where it belongs.

You have the responsibility for your feelings, too. You need not take charge of any other feelings but your own. You should care that others suffer, but realize that you cannot order their feelings. Be considerate of others but maintain your healthful self-responsibility and integrity. You really are growing tall and strong, aren't you?

What have you done right today? You firmly rejected manipulative attempts to make you change. You see that you are in charge of your own feelings.

Today's Action Plan: I will reject attempts to make me responsible for feelings other than my own. I will guard against others' demands which lead to overeating.

You Can Think What You Want

*He who asks of life nothing but the improvement of his
own nature is less liable than anyone else
to miss and waste life.*
Henri Frederic Amiel

Here's a hot bulletin. You are a fabulous storehouse of
valuable resources! Even if your life is beset with problems and you're at the end of your rope, you can still
hang on and win. Why? Because your storehouse of
courage won't let you fall. Just the fact that you read
these words this minute marks you as a special person,
someone who has not quit. Did you know that?

You can solve more problems and hang on longer
because you know you can.

You can't become what you don't believe. If you
believe you can achieve, you're halfway to success. Now
put your confidence in Action, and win.

Negative thinking is an expensive habit; you pay with
your life. You just putter around, nibbling away at your
life, never achieving what you can be.

Half a life is not for you. Move out front and earn
everything you think is wonderful. No one will give it to
you, but you can give it to yourself. But first, get food
out of your way with right-eating, get your body
energized and moving with your choice of exercise, and
digest the Action MindSteps to change the way you feel
about yourself. Take a big bite out of life, won't you?

What have you done right today? You recognized that
you have the resource of courage. You will succeed only
by believing you can.

Today's Action Plan: I will plan how I want to act. I
will act the way I plan.

September 23

Your Belief System

It is impossible to predict what is not possible.
Author unknown

Be careful what you wish for, warns an old saying, you might get it. That's more true if you act on your wish. Your "belief system" is your actions directed by your feelings, thoughts, and attitudes. So if you want something you don't have — thinness, for example — you must change the way you feel, think, and act. You can see that, can't you?

You have the potential to become what your Action MindStep belief system dictates. Your positive inner force, powered by desires, pushes you toward health and confident attitudes. You may not realize it, but you desire MindStep changes. When you overate, you were bored, dull, lifeless. But you wished to lose weight.

Predict thinness and shut out all contrary feelings and attitudes. Each day your positive, winning belief system stimulates you to grow toward your desire of a thin, energized body and a confident self-respect.

Your old belief system doesn't matter today. Your age and weight goal don't matter. Your new belief system, grounded in the Twelve Action MindSteps, will take you where you want to go. Believe that, won't you?

What have you done right today? You saw that your feelings, thoughts, and attitudes formed your belief system. You have adopted the Action MindStep system to get the winning life you wished for.

Today's Action Plan: I will adjust my belief system to help me become what I want to be. I will predict thinness.

The Halo Effect

The anticipation of failure is a self-fulfilling prophecy.
Author unknown

Determining one's whole personality from a single char-
acteristic results in what some psychologists call a "halo
effect." Some overeaters think this way. They fared
badly on a diet once, and they expect diets to go badly
again and again in the same circumstances. Anticipation
of failure can be a self-fulfilling prophecy for overeaters
who say, "I always fall off my diet at restaurants." You
see how the halo effect works against your best interests,
don't you?

The chain can be broken. If you have a negative
experience, learn from it. Learning is a form of success
which you can immediately reinforce.

Keep a record of the lessons you learn from a negative
experience. Anyone can be angry or hopeless or quit
because of a bad experience. It's easy to say, "I won't do
that again, because it never works."

You're not one of the "never" people. If you fall, you
get up, learn the lesson, and go on to do it well the next
time. You break negative chains, don't you?

What have you done right today? You learned that
the halo effect projects a chain reaction of failure into the
future, making it come true. You broke the chain.

**Today's Action Plan: I will not let one failure dictate
to me. I will break the chain of failure by learning what
went wrong.**

September 25

Which Road to Follow

[Cheshire Cat says] " . . . it doesn't matter which way
you go."
" . . . so long as I get somewhere," Alice adds.
"Oh, you're sure to do that," says the Cat, "if you only
walk long enough."

Lewis Carroll

And so it is with so many overweight people (thin ones, too). If you don't know or care where you're going, any road will take you there. If you have no goal, you don't know where you're going or which road to follow. Do you know which road to follow?

Set a specific goal. "I want to lose weight" is not specific. "I want to lose 37-1/2 pounds," is specific.

Your weight goal must be positive. "I don't want to be fat and ugly" is not a positive goal. "I want to lose weight so that I will be happy, healthy, and more attractive" is a positive goal.

You see the difference. You don't want to flounder for the rest of your life. You care where you're going, right? You have a choice between something and nothing. You know your goal. Now climb up the Twelve Action MindSteps to self-respect and success. That's a great way to get somewhere, isn't it?

What have you done right today? You set specific, positive weight and living goals. Today you dug deeper and reached higher than you once thought you could. You are on the MindStep climb to success.

Today's Action Plan: I will care where I'm going. I will have a goal and a way to reach it.

Achieving Goals

Laboring toward distant aims sets the mind in a higher key and puts us at our best.

C. H. Parkhurst

The primary objectives of this book are to help you set your life goals and put you on the right road to achieve them. Of course you have many personal goals unique to your life and circumstances. But you have three goals in common with every other reader of this book: you want to control your weight, you want to re-energize your body so you will have the vitality to achieve your goals, and you want to view life as winners do. Isn't that so?

There are criteria for achieving goals in right-eating, exercise, and in following the Action MindSteps. They are:

1. Set a specific, positive goal.
2. Provide effective motivation with interim goals.
3. Develop continuous effort; regularity is the key.
4. Overcome setbacks by learning from problems.
5. Recognize and celebrate small successes.

What is your goal? Make a plan for achieving it today. You will never have to say, "I wish I had." Postponing is a waste of your life, isn't it?

What have you done right today? You decided on an goal and developed a plan for achieving it. You're not standing in line with your hand out. You're in charge. That's a good day's work!

Today's Action Plan: I will set goals for myself. I will not waste my life by postponing Action.

Have You Got a Hunch?

A hunch is creativity trying to tell you something.
Anonymous

You've broken through the debilitating cycle of overeat-starve-overeat through understanding and Action. You are developing a strong sense of yourself — "ego strength," psychologists call it. You have a hunch that something good is happening to you, haven't you?

Your life is now built around a central idea — a solid understanding of your self-worth. You know that you deserve to achieve your goals, to become a thinner winner.

Aimless overeating formerly dissipated your energy, fatigued, and bored you. Today, playing life to win, you are alive, joyous, and vital.

You were born to be happy, healthy, and successful. But you looked for happiness in food when it was within you all the time. Seek within yourself. You are not at the mercy of food or happenstance. You have all that you need to be a winner.

Overeating once subtracted from your happy, autonomous living, but now you are in charge of your eating and your life. It's exciting to take charge of your life, to find you have a will of your own. Doing what needs to be done promptly is a basic part of rational living, and your life makes sense now, doesn't it?

What have you done right today? You have a hunch that your life is going to be wonderful, and you're right.

Today's Action Plan: I will pay attention to my positive hunches. I will build my life on a solid understanding of my unique worth.

September 28

Just Your Luck!

I think luck is the sense to recognize an opportunity and the ability to take advantage of it. Everyone has bad breaks, but everyone also has opportunities.

Samuel Goldwyn

Do you see every bump in the road as an example of your bad luck? "Just my luck!" you say when something goes awry. This attitude is a subtle form of self-sabotage. Do you know why?

Look again at the words, "Just *my* luck!" You are equating your luck with your self-worth, as though your luck would be better if *you* were better. With that attitude you'll see every evidence of bad luck as proof of your own unworthiness. You can see how destructive such thinking is, can't you?

Face facts! Luck has nothing to do with your weight. Luck is an opportunity you either take advantage of, or don't. For that matter, you hold a lucky opportunity in your hand. Will you take advantage of what you read here and apply it to your weight and living problems? Say YES.

Make your own luck. Today is a gift, an opportunity to continue improving your life. You're a lucky person, do you know that?

What have you done right today? You realized that thinking you are singled out for bad luck is a negative game you played with your self-worth.

Today's Action Plan: I will see opportunities as luck. I will take advantage of my lucky day.

September 29

Use Your Momentum for Change

There are no permanent changes because change itself is permanent.

Ralph L. Woods

Most diet experts warn against trying to change other habits while you're losing weight. This may be good advice when you are just beginning weight control, or if a diet is merely added to your present life. But other changes are possible when right-eating is integrated as part of a LifeWay system. You are proof of that, aren't you?

You've already changed from sedentary habits to physical exercise, and changed your low self-esteem to high regard.

One overweight who had lost seventy pounds said, "I felt so strong and confident, with energy to spare, that I quit smoking before I'd lost all my weight."

You, too, can use the momentum you have gained from your three-part living plan to tackle other changes you want to make — quit smoking, reduce alcohol consumption, change jobs, go back to school, move to another locale, and so on.

Once you're truly on the road to achieving a thinner body, you can continue to make good changes. You're ready, aren't you?

What have you done right today? You used the momentum and strength and confidence of your take-charge program to make good changes in your life.

Today's Action Plan: I will make other good changes after I have overeating under control. I see change as a challenge.

September 30

Back to Basics

*If we search for the fundamentals which actually moti-
vate us, we will find . . . it is to some of them that we
owe that big urge which pushes us onward.*
Edward S. Jordan

The best educators return to school for refresher courses.
The great professional athletes still take coaching lessons
on fundamental moves and strategy. The most talented
concert pianists continue to practice their keyboard
exercises. That's true, isn't it?

All these people, tops in their fields, have something in
common. They realize that one must maintain the basics,
the solid foundation of fundamentals on which success
was built.

Recovering overeaters, too, must maintain a solid
foundation of fundamentals. You know what they are:
your right-eating food plan, regular exercise, and a
positive attitude; your twelve Action MindSteps to give
you strength and direction; and these pages to motivate
and help you get started each day. These are the tested
basics you need to be a winner, aren't they?

What have you done right today? You went back to
basics for a refresher course. Like all champions, you
know that fundamentals help you keep winning.

**Today's Action Plan: I will never get far from the
fundamentals on which my new LifeWay is built. When
I have a problem, I will first determine what basic self-
respectful truth I am not following.**

Diet Groups Are Not for All

I felt smothered by people who wanted too much of me, and who, because I had lost weight, thought I owed them everything.

Diet group member

Diet groups help a great many people lose weight, but they're not for everyone. Membership in any group means loss of some individuality, some freedom to think, feel, and act for ourselves. If the advantages — a supportive environment, more self-understanding, learning more about your weight problem — are greater than the disadvantages, you'll be content. If not, you'll need to look further, won't you?

Visit a variety of weight-losing groups. Ask yourself these questions before deciding on one: Do you get understanding? Is the group too expensive? Do you see success? Does the group withdraw friendship from those who slip off the prescribed diet? Does the group attack, or encourage? Is the group immature and full of squabbling? Does the group have a pedestal complex, raising successful members up and later knocking them down?

Even the best group may not be for you. Or you may want to attend meetings occasionally to boost your spirits. Whatever you decide is right. You're in charge, aren't you?

What have you done right today? You have a checklist to evaluate weight-loss groups. You see that you can join a group and go regularly, occasionally, or not at all. As it is with everything in your life, the choice is yours.

Today's Action Plan: I will evaluate groups carefully. I will make choices that decrease frustration and increase contentment.

The Big Difference

Many people go from infancy to senility without ever achieving maturity.

Anonymous

The big difference between immaturity and maturity, between dependence and independence, between a loser and a winner, is self-understanding. Most of us overeaters are confused about self-understanding. We call it "self-awareness," using the two terms interchangeably. The terms are as different as day and night, green and pink, an adolescent girl and a grandmother, and it's a crucial difference. That's clear, isn't it?

Self-awareness is a game we play with ourselves and others. It shows everybody how much we know about ourselves, how sensitive and psychologically sophisticated we are. But it's a loser's game unless it progresses to self-understanding. Here's the difference. Self-awareness merely says, "I know why I hurt!" Self-understanding bravely says, "This is my mess and I must clean it up myself."

Maturity is independence; independence is maturity. Say it any way you want, the results are the same. To be dependent on our hurts without taking responsibility for them and putting them right is to spend life in a helpless dither. You don't want that, do you?

What have you done right today? You have discovered the difference between self-awareness and self-understanding. Because you have a goal in life, you have seen that it's not enough just to be aware of your feelings. The big difference between you and a loser is that you are going to do something about your feelings.

Today's Action Plan: I will not say "I hurt" without finding a way to stop hurting. I will take charge of my awareness.

"No Excuse, Sir."

The difficult we do immediately — the impossible takes a little longer.
Slogan of the United States Army Corps of Engineers

Anyone who served in the military knows that alibis for failure to perform are frowned on by superior officers. The only acceptable explanation is, "No excuse, sir." Even if you have a good excuse, it's considered inappropriate to offer it. It takes a lot of self-confidence not to offer an excuse if you have one, doesn't it?

Self-confidence is another name for security. Practice it. Stop making excuses for possible failure in your program of right-eating, exercise, and Action MindSteps. Instead, find reasons why you will succeed.

If you're not sure you can do great things, remember: when you're not overeating today, you're doing what was impossible yesterday.

Don't get stuck in the trap of past pain. What overeating did to you isn't as important as what you do about your overeating.

Succeed today. Then search for the clues to your success so you can use them again. Now isn't that self-affirming and powerful?

What have you done right today? You see that taking total responsibility for your Actions is the most confident thing you can do. You are a good soldier.

Today's Action Plan: I will make no excuses. I will not overeat today, doing today what was impossible yesterday.

Positive Rewards

Learn to repeat endlessly to yourself: 'It all depends on me.'

André Gide

Success is setting and attaining goals. You believe that already, don't you? The question is how you can insure that you will repeat the positive behavior that brings you physical and mental fitness. Rewarding yourself can do wonders. Would you like to hear more?

You know that we tend to repeat behavior which brings positive feedback. But did you know we are most apt to repeat behavior that brings us *immediate* positive feedback? (Food can do that; our senses of smell, sight and touch are immediately engaged.)

Today you want immediate reinforcements for your new way of healthful eating. How? Make a list of positive reinforcers, non-food items you really enjoy, like a telephone chat with a friend or relative, reading a good book, listening to favorite music.

Keep records of positive eating behavior as a reinforcement. Make a chart and token system. For example, give yourself a token for every day you follow your right-eating plan. When you amass a certain number of tokens (you decide how many), give yourself an extra-special reward, maybe new clothes, theater tickets, or a trip. The idea is to reinforce success immediately so you will continue to do what will lead to the biggest reward, your new body and life. You like the idea of immediate positive rewards, don't you?

What have you done right today? You fed yourself positive reinforcement instead of extra food. There is nothing more right for you to do today.

Today's Action Plan: I will give my right-eating plan immediate positive reinforcement. I will believe that right-eating depends on me.

October 5

Unfinished Business

To be what we are, and to become what we are capable of becoming, is the only end of life.
Robert Louis Stevenson

When you overate, life was so stressful that you were continually off balance. It's as if one hand (your desire to stop) pushed against the other (your compulsion to overeat). What is the unfinished business of your life? What are the things you most want to do? Now that you have a plan, a LifeWay, you can imagine yourself doing them. When you control your eating, you are better able to control other events in your life. You can get on to unfinished business, can't you?

"O to be self-balanced . . . ," wrote Walt Whitman. You know the joy of having your life in balance, having your goals agree with what your mind tells you to do. You found a way to take risks so you are challenged, but not so many that you are overwhelmed. You mastered the tug and pull between playing it safe and driving for success. You know the difference between the false and temporary fullness after overeating and the real fullness of right-eating.

With overeating out of the way, you can begin to tackle the unfinished business of your life. Do it today, won't you?

What have you done right today? You know the difference between the stressful imbalance of the overeater's life and the security of your right-eating, exercise, and MindStep attitudes. You wouldn't trade your new life for anything.

Today's Action Plan: I will get on with any unfinished business in my life. I will be master of what I eat.

October 6

Happiness Re-examined

Happiness is the only sanction of life; where happiness fails, existence remains a mad, lamentable experiment.
                                                              Santayana

Life has no meaning without happiness or at least some hope of attaining it. Like the old joke says, happiness is no laughing matter. It is both joyful and profoundly serious. You've discovered that, haven't you?

For overeaters there can be little happiness when eating is out of control. In the past, we lived with dissatisfaction, instability, criticism, boredom, helplessness, and under-utilization of our abilities. When we overate, happiness failed.

But when you chose right-eating, exercise, and Action MindStep attitudes, the road ahead became smooth. A happy life became possible. Should you reach even half your happiness potential, you'll do better than most people. And you, of all these people, have the best chance to attain all the happiness you deserve. How could this be? Because you are capable of compulsion — so far, misdirected toward food — which you can translate into drive. Paradoxically, the very trait that got you into trouble can make you a winner, if you turn it toward achievement. Now you hunger for success, and the happiness that goes with it. Isn't that true?

What have you done right today? You found where your true happiness lies and you are going to give it your all, plus 10 percent.

Today's Action Plan: I will never return to the hell of overeating. I will drive forward to happiness.

October 7

Diet-group Dropout Guilt

It was a real Catch-22 situation. I was unhappy with my diet group, but I was afraid if I didn't keep going, I'd regain all my weight.

Ex-diet-group member

You should give a group a chance to help you, since so many overeaters find success in self-help diet groups. But if you become unhappy with a group for any reason, you have a perfect right to leave. Despite any dire predictions, do not *expect* to regain your lost weight. If you believe you are helpless working alone, you run the risk of fulfilling the group's prophecy, don't you?

First of all, when you join a group tell yourself you will stay or leave as you choose. Later, if you decide to withdraw, do so without guilt or fear. Here are four ways to ease the strain of leaving:

1. Choose a time when you're having success in your life, other than weight loss.
2. Announce your plan to leave ahead of time so you can say good-bye. You don't have to sneak out.
3. Use your powerful, positive vocabulary. Rather than "dropping out" from failure, you are "graduating" after success.
4. Believe that you have the right to continue weight-loss independently, and the right to come back to the group later, if you choose.

You have every right to make free choices, don't you?

What have you done right today? You know that you are in charge of your life. You make the choices and accept the responsibility.

Today's Action Plan: I will never stay in a diet group out of fear. I make my own choices and live without guilt.

Believe How Good You Are

Stature comes not with height but with depth.
Benjamin Lichtenberg

You are a person of value, a good deal better than you think you are. The inner you is not negative, and you're no quitter. Today you are positive and a winner. Believe that. The real you does not lack for brains and courage. Believe that too, won't you?

Don't be discouraged today or any day, even if you fall short of your capabilities. You are human. When you are less than you know you can be, less than you want to be, be gentle with yourself. Then get to work again. The real you is inherently patient, kind, forgiving, warmly caring, dependable, and strong. Believe that.

You needn't wait until your body is slender to accept your goodness. You needn't put off enjoying a new LifeWay of healthful eating, exercise, and attitudes until you are more deserving; you deserve it now.

Cooperate with your good. Be sympathetic with yourself. Everything you want to be will take root. Believe that, won't you? Nod YES.

What have you done right today? You accepted the fact that you are a valuable person, but human. You don't expect to falter, but if you do, you will be sympathetic with yourself, and get right back into Action.

Today's Action Plan: I will believe my inner good. I will look for good in myself and work on the rest.

Recreate Your Body

I believe the potential for (physical) transformation is available to every . . . human being.
Dr. Suki Rappaport

You are always recreating, always changing your body. Think about that. You are physically different from five years or even a year ago. Every second, 2.5 million red blood cells are created and die in your body. What kind of body are you recreating today?

Can you channel physical change in the direction you'd like it to go? You bet you can! Cooperate with your body. It wants and needs health. It is transformed with right-eating, physical exercise, and your glowing new attitudes.

Overeating is life-threatening. That doesn't mean that overeating, unless it's tragically out of control, will kill you. It does mean that overeating threatens to keep you from living fully, even from feeling completely alive.

Create a vivid image in your mind of the body you want to begin creating today. Use this image to reinforce your three-part living plan. Then follow this image with Action. You have the power to transform your body totally. Do you have an image of how you will look? Beautiful!

What have you done right today? You see that you have the power to literally grow a new body day by day. Your self-image is of a whole, strong, beautiful body.

Today's Action Plan: I will eat to recreate the body I want. I will exercise, and live by my new, winning attitudes.

The Will to Win

*If you have the will to win, you have achieved half your
success; if you don't, you have achieved
half your failure.*
David V. A. Ambrose

Overweights seldom commit physical suicide. But too
many of us commit a little mental suicide. We throw up
our hands and say, "I just can't go on." That's a pretty
extreme feeling, isn't it?

Surveys of how people feel about themselves show
that overweights are less happy with themselves than
thinner people. Of course they're unhappy about their
weight, but surprisingly that's not the root of their
unhappiness. They feel a lack of control over themselves.
Do you know what a hopeless feeling that is?

We humans have little control over circumstances
outside ourselves. Weather, war, economic depression —
all are beyond our individual sway. But if we feel we
have no influence, even over ourselves, we feel completely helpless and powerless.

You will be unhappy to the extent that you feel out-of-
control. Take charge of what you eat today. It is the
most important thing you can do for yourself. Without
eating-control, nothing can follow. With eating-control,
everything falls into place. It's about time you put
happiness into your life, isn't it?

What have you done right today? You faced the
reason for your unhappiness. Every day, your right-
eating plan is leading to the happy life.

**Today's Action Plan: I will not kill my chance for
happiness by overeating. I know that good will follow
from self-control.**

Headed in the Right Direction

Go confidently in the direction of your dreams. Live the life you have imagined.
Henry David Thoreau

These pages will help you to become your own agent for change. Change needs direction — your direction. Only you know what you want. Only you have the power to take yourself there. As always, the paramount change for you is to get overeating out of the way so you can find what your life is meant to be. Surely you are not on this earth to be just an eating machine. That is not the life you imagine, is it?

Today, as every day, your first serious mental act is to review your chosen LifeWay and the eating, exercising, attitude changes you have made. Ask yourself a series of questions:

1. "What is my problem?" Assess your eating problem (or any other).
2. "How does it make me feel or act?" Assess food's negative power.
3. "What can I do about it?" Make your decision for today.
4. "Will I do it?" Make your commitment for today.
5. "How will I achieve it?" Evaluate and improve your plan.

Because of the choices you make right now, you are no longer just an eating machine; you are more truly yourself. It's true, isn't it?

What have you done right today? You chose to be in charge of your life's direction.

Today's Action Plan: I will set my own course. I will live my life as I imagined I would.

Stop, Damned Thought!

*Unless a capacity for thinking be accompanied by a
capacity for action, a superior mind exists in torture.*
                                        Benedetto Croce

Are you, despite your best efforts, sometimes haunted by
thoughts of certain foods? That's not unusual. When you
are tired, hungry, frustrated, the old ways of dealing
with these feelings can sneak back into your mind. Has
that ever happened to you?

Remember you're the food boss, so you're in charge.
Practice stopping food thoughts.

Visualize yourself in a mindscape of foods which
sometimes obsess you. Develop this scene cinematically;
add color, costumes, dramatic effects, lighting. See your
hand reaching for the food. Shout, "Stop!" Replace the
scene with the image of you, slender, running like the
wind on a country road on a crisp autumn morning.

Repeat the thought-stopping technique until you can
shift from a sudden desire for certain foods to an image
of you as you want to be. With practice, you can
become so adept that you can change thoughts at will.

As a problem-solver, you must know what your mind
is doing and how to reprogram it for a winning LifeWay.
Food fantasies are destructive for you. What you do is
reality; and reality, not fantasy, is your friend. You
agree, don't you?

What have you done right today? You learned a
technique to stop obsessive thoughts of food. You
replaced a negative thought with the image of your real
self.

**Today's Action Plan: I will practice stopping negative
thoughts. I will take charge of my food obsession.**

October 13

Cold-weather Exercise Addicts

*After eight to ten weeks . . . you'll find yourself looking
forward to your exercise, longing for it
as an accustomed pleasure.*
Dr. Kenneth H. Cooper

By including daily physical exercise in your weight-
control program, you have become devoted to it. So you
really feel deprived when bad weather keeps you from
exercise and fun. Don't despair! Switch to indoor exercise. Even if you're housebound, there are physical
activities which will maintain weight loss and keep you
feeling alive. Continue moving, won't you?

Try stationary running on a thick carpet. Use up-
tempo music if you need help maintaining a steady
rhythm.

Try skipping rope. (Maybe it helped keep you trim as
a youngster.) There's an advantage to rope-skipping over
running in place. It adds tone to muscles in your arms,
shoulders, and chest. Not a bad pay-off for a few
minutes a day.

Three-step climbing is another easy, first-rate indoor
exercise. Up and down three steps for five munutes can
give you maximum aerobic benefits. What could be
simpler?

Combine and vary these indoor exercises to maintain
the wonderful sense of physical self you've developed
through your three-part LifeWay. You really want to go
right on feeling great, don't you? Say YES, and jump for
joy.

What have you done right today? You found a way to
continue your physical program, no matter what the
weather is like outside. You no longer look for reasons
to quit, but ways to continue.

Today's Action Plan: I will plan indoor exercise for
inclement weather. I will do the exercises and have fun
doing them.

Overeating Is Boring

*I never went anywhere, never did anything new. I just
wanted everybody to get out of my way,
so I could eat, eat, eat!*
Member of Overeaters Anonymous

Too little has been written in how-to-lose-weight books
— and too little is known by experts — about the
chronic, awful boredom of an overeater's life. When we
become involved totally with food, we shut out everything and everyone. We may not tell others to go away
and leave us alone, but that's what we feel, and they
must sense our feelings. Do you understand how this
could happen?

It's boring to spend time hiding in the bathroom
because you've hidden candy bars in the hamper.

It's boring to explain for the tenth time that your new
diet will take time to show results.

It's boring to be scared to death of the medical clinic
scale, the look on the nurse's face, and the disappointment in your doctor's eyes.

Overeating created a continuing crisis in your life —
and even that was boring.

Today you have a program of right-eating, exercise,
and MindStep attitudes that brings you more excitement
than overeating ever could. Your new LifeWay is ever-
changing. You are fantastically alive! There is no way
you could stand the boredom of overeating again, is
there?

What have you done right today? You saw how
exciting your life has become now that you play life to
win.

Today's Action Plan: I will never return to the awful
boredom of living to eat. Today I chose the ever-
changing excitement of Action MindStep living.

October 15

You Are Free to Choose

Man's last freedom is his freedom to choose . . .
Viktor Frankl

You don't have to live in an underprivileged country or in a big-city ghetto to have a poor quality of life. Overeaters know they can make a food-prison out of a mansion. That's true, isn't it?

When you embraced the Action attitudes of the Twelve Action MindSteps, you created a comfort zone for yourself. No matter where or how you live, there is a circle of comfort surrounding you. That is why it is important that every former overeater learn to make changes whenever necessary to insure continued right-eating.

Although overeaters are alike in many ways, each is unique, too. You have your own needs, you live in your own way, and your work, family, and social setting are not the same as other overeaters!

Taking charge of your life is a process of making choices, discovering what works for you. This is the continuing, exciting challenge of your life.

No one is closer to the core of your being than you are. No one else can make informed choices for your life better than you can. In the end, all choice is yours, all responsibility, all victory. You wouldn't have it any other way, would you?

What have you done right today? You added a fresh appreciation for the rich diversity of choices you can make for your life. This is a freedom you've always wanted.

Today's Action Plan: I will take charge of the quality of my life. Through good choices, I will make a palace of my prison.

October 16

The Big Put-off

Indecision is debilitating; it feeds upon itself . . . . [You]
are dependent upon action. [You] cannot go forward by
hesitation. Often greater risk is involved
in postponement than in making a wrong decision.

H. A. Hopf

"I'm going to stop overeating, and this time I really mean
it!" Sounds final, doesn't it?

Even this courageous announcement is still just so
many words — positively stated, it's true — but just a
wish. What happened when, despite your vow, you
overate in the middle of the morning? Did you set off a
chain reaction of procrastination?

After you overate, you berated yourself. Instead of
making a new beginning right on the spot, you postponed. Next you defended your behavior. "After all,"
you said, "I've already slipped. No sense starting over
today. I already blew the whole diet, didn't I?"

So you spent the day overeating, using food to cover
up your dislike for what you did. You were terribly
uneasy all day. Next morning, you assured yourself you
wouldn't procrastinate again. Days and weeks, months
and years pass in a blur of such broken promises, food
binges, and tearful regrets.

Had enough of times like those? You bet you have!
You took the Action MindStep road out of that hell.
Now you have a direction and a plan in your life. You're
a winner. Aren't you glad it's today and not the old
days?

What have you done right today? You decided that
never again will you only vow to stop overeating. You
traded broken vows for Action.

Today's Action Plan: I will not play a losing game
with procrastination. I will play life to win.

The Game of Pretend

*At last, I can be myself. I don't have to make things look
good on the outside while I'm dying on the inside.*
Diet workshop participant

Overeaters living in a thin-is-right, fat-is-wrong society
usually play three roles. The *happy clown* role says,
"Everything's wonderful!" The *sad clown* role says, "Pity
poor me!" The *flippant clown* role says, "I don't care!"
Overweights play so many roles they lose their real
selves. Were you one of these?

Did you try to make things look good on the outside,
while feeling bad on the inside? Did you work hard
maintaining the "happy clown" facade and denying your
true feelings of helplessness. Did you often wonder if
overeating was worth it?

Did you feel so rotten on the inside that you *wanted*
others to know and pity you? Did you feel you had to
deny that you get any pleasure from life at all? Did you
often wonder if overeating was worth it?

Did you build an "I don't care" image and behave as if
you believed it? Did you deny that you wanted other
people to like you? Did you often wonder if overeating
was worth it?

Now that you have found your new LifeWay, you
have the answer. Overeating is *not* worth it! You know
you become who you truly are when you stop overeating. You know that food gets in your way, smothers and
distorts every emotion. You know you want to follow
your right-eating, exercise and Action MindSteps. You
know who your real self is, and you like the new,
honest, guilt-free person you have become, don't you?

What have you done right today? You put away your
repertoire of false clown roles. Who is that coming this
way? Why, it's you!

Today's Action Plan: I will bring the curtain down on
all false self-images. I will begin to find my true self.

Growing

*The more we can control our anxiety and reduce its
crippling effects, the more we can make positive use of it
in our striving to understand, accept, tolerate, and
respect ourselves and others.*
Henry Clay Lindgren

Do you welcome change? Growing, making positive
changes, is emotionally healthy. The alternative is decay,
because people, like societies, don't stand still. You can
believe that, can't you?

A basic law of nature is that living things strive
against all odds to grow. Embryos in mothers' wombs
continue to mature unless they are prevented from
growing by physical problems.

When you overeat, you are in conflict with life's
physical law of healthful growth. Excess food stifles your
innate drive toward complete development. It's an obstacle you can't get over or around on the way to fulfilling
your potential.

Overeating must be eliminated before you can reach
emotional maturity, and maturity is only one of the
pleasures of growth. Add it to the list of other pleasurable achievements like low anxiety, enhanced talents, and
satisfying relationships. You deserve to grow toward
your full potential. You've made a good start. Keep on,
won't you?

What have you done right today? You welcomed the
idea of positive change, so you can grow toward your
full potential.

**Today's Action Plan: I will rid myself of excess food
so I can be all I was meant to be. I will continue to grow
emotionally.**

There's So Much in You

*Every one to whom much is given,
of him much will be required.*

Luke 12:48

There are so many overeaters struggling with food compulsion who can barely tolerate themselves. It's so sad, because they've been given so much. Read on, won't you?

You were given a brain for clear thinking and wise judgment. Excess food dimmed your ability to think positively, but didn't extinguish it.

You were given courage and strength to withstand the problems of living in a rapidly changing world. Overeating kept you from using your courageous spirit to help yourself.

You were given heightened senses which became blurred by bingeing and dulled the shine on your emotional life.

You had all that it took to reach success. Only one obstacle stood in your way — overeating.

You've always had everything necessary to make your life work better. And today you are making wise eating and exercise decisions, and using the MindSteps to power yourself into Action. Now you're in charge of your life. Now you are using what you have been given to make wonderful changes. It's a grand day, isn't it?

What have you done right today? You took stock of the wonderful abilities you've been given. You are using them to make a winning change in your life.

Today's Action Plan: I will use the abilities I've been given. I will get rid of the one obstacle that stands in my way — overeating.

Reflection

As one thinketh in his heart, so is he.

Proverbs 23:7

Get quiet. At least once a day go to a place where you can hear the silence, where you will be able to listen to your inner voices without any distractions. There are so many demands for your attention today — television, family, friends, work. Sometimes, you can go for weeks without any quiet time alone. You're ready to listen now, aren't you?

Understanding who you are, getting to know your own wants, demand time and the proper atmosphere for reflection. You don't have to go to a mountain top or a deserted beach (although water is soothing), but it will help to get as far from interference as possible.

A quiet walk, a few minutes of solitude, a momentary vacation in a tranquil corner, will give you a much-needed respite from the tension-producing "everyday-ness" of life. Even winners must rest and learn to listen to their minds and bodies. You wouldn't want to miss an important message because you weren't listening, would you?

What have you done right today? You have granted yourself the peace of a few minutes out of your hectic day. Getting away from it all, you have learned, is one way you maintain a high performance level. Do it, because you've earned it.

Today's Action Plan: I will give myself a few minutes of my time. I will concentrate on the first Action MindStep, understanding my unique worth.

October 21

Worst Case Scenario

*There are days when it takes all you've got
just to keep up . . .*

Robert Orben

Some days you're faced with puzzling choices. Should
you take this job or that one; move to the country or
stay in the city. Those are the diet days when you're
tempted to say, "Oh, the heck with it." Be careful. At
times like this it's easy to slip back into the quagmire of
stuffing food into the bottomless pit of indecision.
You've fallen into this trap before, haven't you?

Why not try decision-making using a worst case
scenario? If you take the new job, or move to the
country, what's the worst thing that could happen? You
could lose money or hate the country. Then what's the
worst thing that could happen? You could go broke or
move back to the city. What terrible thing might happen
then? You could get a new job or try to relocate in your
old neighborhood. You can go on with this game but
you get the idea. When you've made a bad choice, the
worst thing that can happen is that you'll be faced with
more choices. What's the best thing that can happen?
Each time you choose, you learn.

But remember that choice is only possible if you are in
control of your eating. One of the hidden consequences
of overeating is to remove your decision-making abilities. Isn't that so?

What have you done right today? A day may begin
with puzzling choices, but if you act rather than eat
you'll never be at the mercy of happenstance.

**Today's Action Plan: I will not be trapped into
overeating by indecision. I will be in charge of my
choices.**

October 22

Double Reward

*The effects of our actions may be postponed but they are
never lost. There is an inevitable reward for good deeds
and an inescapable punishment for bad. Meditate upon
this truth, and seek always to earn good wages from
Destiny.*

Wu Ming Fu

Throughout this book you have been reading a life-
changing motivational phrase: *Do today what you know
you want to do.* These are deceptively simple words,
with a life-saving message. It tells overeaters: when you
don't do what you need and want to do, you come into
immediate conflict with your own conscience. You
believe that, don't you?

There is a double reward for doing what you know
you need to do. First, you feel worthwhile, not in
conflict with your basic belief. Second, the job gets done.
For overeaters this means building self-esteem and losing
excess weight too. These are big rewards for pleasing
yourself, aren't they?

Don't grab for the momentary pleasure of overeating,
but for deeper rewards. Don't settle for the moment's
indulgence when you can have the double reward of self-
esteem and a thinner body. Doesn't two-for-the-price-of-
one make better sense?

What have you done right today? You earned the
good wages of destiny by doing what you know you
need to do for your body, mind, and emotions. That's a
smart move.

Today's Action Plan: I will multiply my rewards as I
subtract pounds by doing what I know needs to be done.
I will grab for real future rewards rather than a momentary food indulgence.

October 23

If

If you can . . . start again at your beginnings and never breathe a word about your loss.

Rudyard Kipling

Remember that time you lost a lot of weight? You were filled with joy. Life would be different — better, you thought. You would never again be overweight. But you got careless; Action disappeared from your days, and then you started to slip. The pounds came back fast, didn't they?

What are you saying right now? "Not me! This time when I lose weight, I won't forget how I did it." But you will, unless you and the Action ideas are one, unless they become part of you and you become part of them. If you remember only one thing from these pages, remember that. Don't downgrade the Action techniques which helped you achieve your weight loss. Keep doing what produced results.

Build discipline into your life. Discipline is a concept that has fallen among bad companions in the past few decades. It's supposed to inhibit personal freedom, dry up creativity, and smother spontaneity. But for overeaters, discipline is a life-saver. You need an anchor, truth, commitment. You need structure in your life, don't you?

What have you done right today? You have recognized the trap in forgetting your Action plan. Don't change what works!

Today's Action Plan: I will build structure into my life. I will take hold of the Action principles and never let them go.

October 24

The Magic Hand from the Past

*More powerful is he who has himself
in his own power.*

Seneca

You say, "She eats candy bars and never gains an ounce. I just *look* at sweets and put on ten pounds." And didn't your mother make you clean your plate? And doesn't your mate complain about waste? And don't your friends tempt you with fresh-baked goodies? Damn! No wonder you're overweight. It's all their fault, isn't it?

It can be momentarily satisfying to play "poor baby," but it's an irresponsible way to live. Fat is not a rotten thing other people do to you. No matter what your mother told you as a child, if you're still cleaning your plate (and everyone else's) as an adult, you're making your own choices.

There is no magic hand from the past controlling your fork.

Blaming others for what we do is both aggressive and passive. "I'll show them what they did to me!" and "Poor me, there's nothing I can do once I've been programmed this way."

Haven't you suffered long enough from the "magic hand"? Take charge of your life and the food in your life. It is the only way, isn't it?

What have you done right today? You saw that the "poor baby" game is one you can't win. You took responsibility for your own eating. Now you can take Action.

Today's Action Plan: I will take charge of the food in my life. I will be an achieving adult, not a victim of my past.

See Success

To try and to fail is at least to learn; to fail to try is to suffer the inestimable loss of what might have been.
                                                    Chester Barnard

Eating something not on your right-eating plan doesn't mean you've lost everything. If you have been eating right for a week — for twenty-one meals — and you overeat at one meal, you didn't "blow the whole week." Don't see only failures; see successes instead. Learn to see the twenty successes you had, and you will not lose perspective on that single overeating episode. This is the true balance you're searching for, isn't it?

Let's say you set a weight goal and haven't reached it yet. Don't look at this and see yourself as a failure. You're not a rotten person just because you didn't reach a goal by a certain time.

Accept your humanness. Saints don't make mistakes, but humans do. Your way is no longer the all-or-nothing way of the frantic overeater or the frantic dieter. You choose a positive, balanced perspective where successes are recognized, and a stumble is something to learn from. This LifeWay is so much better, isn't it?

What have you done right today? You learned to see success as easily as failure. You accepted your humanness. This is the positive way you choose to live your life today and everyday.

Today's Action Plan: I will not let one stumble make me fall back all the way. I wll achieve true balance through a positive perspective.

October 26

Opportunities

*We consume our tomorrows fretting
about our yesterdays.*

Persius

What's gone is gone; what's done is done. To fret over
wasted opportunity means that two opportunities —
yesterday's and today's — have been wasted. Use today
to get ahead of yesterday, not to moan about it. You
want to be too busy living, achieving, and planning to
worry about yesterday's mistakes, don't you?

Repeat this sentence out loud: I choose to say YES to
the opportunities I have because I love each new chance
life gives me.

Seize every new chance to achieve the winning life.
Today you're going to make a difference; you're going to
grab an opportunity, and your heart is going to skip
with excitement.

A person is really living when he or she can say, "I
love where I am this minute, and I will love where I'm
going to be tomorrow." What an optimistic, open,
winning attitude!

Be a person who makes and then seizes opportunity.
Be a winner who cares about good health; stick to your
eating plan; and keep exercising your body. You'll notice
the difference in how you feel about yourself, your life,
and other people. Think about it, won't you? Then do it.

What have you done right today? You have stopped
fretting over yesterday's lost opportunities. You have
become a winner who not only seizes an opportunity,
but who loves to do it. Say, you look thinner already!

**Today's Action Plan: I will forget yesterday's lost
opportunities. I will seize today's chances, and love every
minute of it.**

October 27

Break Out of Negative Habits

*[Behavior change] is not easy — in fact it's damned hard
— but it is possible. That thought's important to me
after so many years of feeling helpless
about my eating.*
Man at a behavior modification workshop

You'd be the first to agree that breaking an overeating
habit isn't easy. During an ordinary day there are so
many places, activities, and emotions that cue you to
eat. And some eating may become so automatic that
sometimes you polish off a no-no before you realize it.
But habit, however strong, is curable. This book is
dedicated to helping you reprogram your destructive
behavior patterns, and to put your new knowledge into
Action. You have no problems with what's been said so
far, have you?

Now you must develop a desirable, positive program.
It's not too late to change the emotional habits that
trigger overeating, nor is it too late to develop an
exercise habit where none existed. Here are guidelines to
help you attain these ends.

1. Know that you can disrupt a negative habit
   pattern (even one of long standing), and
   substitute or create positive new habits.
2. Never scold yourself for having an overeating
   problem. Instead, praise yourself for working
   hard to make a good change in your life.
3. Give yourself enough time to break a habit.
   How many years have you been overeating?
   You deserve as much time to make
   confirmed changes, don't you?

What have you done right today? You found that you
can be in charge of your habits. What a hopeful
discovery!

**Today's Action Plan: I will work at undoing my
destructive habits. I know I can.**

October 28

The High Cost of Diet Fads

It's a pretty corrupt field.
Dr. William I. Bennett

In the United States alone, it is estimated that over 10 billion dollars are spent each year on dieting. England, Germany, Italy, and other countries with sizeable weight problems add billions more pounds, deutschmarks, and lire. How much have you spent on miracle-diet books, pills, or rubber bunny suits?

Most fad diets are nutritionally unbalanced, particularly single-food diets, from brown rice to grapefruit. And so far, no pill has been dicovered that melts fat, blocks starch, or stops food cravings that come from the mind.

The blatant swindles come and go fast, but never disappear from the market. The product name changes, the spiel is updated, and the come-on ads are right back in the media.

Two claims of the fast-buck artists are true. One is that fat is not forever, and second, there *is* a miracle method.

The hucksters have no miracle, but you do. You *are* that miracle ingredient. You and your open, willing mind. You, when you take charge of your life, when you become the director of your own action. No pill, no magic food, no diet-marketeer can do what you can do. Believe this about yourself, won't you?

What have you done right today? You rejected the blatant, cynical attempts to capitalize on your misery. You know that fat is not forever, because you won't allow it.

Today's Action Plan: I will not be mesmerized by promises of diet magic. I will make my own miracle.

Get the Fat Out

Get the fat in your diet to be less than 30 percent of the calories you take in, and everything else falls into line.
Dr. George H. Blackburn

You are in charge of your weight-losing and maintaining plan. Usually it's best to work with a nutritionist, unless you qualify yourself by study. And you can do that. There are a number of understandable texts in your bookstore or library. A good one will help you adjust your caloric intake to a mixture of protein, carbohydrates, and most importantly, 30 percent (or less) mostly unsaturated fats. These are reasonable guidelines, which offer a great deal of choice, aren't they?

Whether you or a nutritionist does the planning, you will want your diet to:

1. Provide a balance of essential vitamins and minerals;
2. Furnish ample food fibers;
3. Deliver weight-loss and weight-control;
4. Fit your way of living;
5. Bring you to optimum health.

Beware of diets that are too low in calories. Radical weight-loss usually means you're just playing water games, losing water, not weight. It can't be said too often: you're in charge of what you eat now. Isn't that a relief?

What have you done right today? You took charge of the food in your life; you are aware of the protein, fat, and carbohydrates in your diet. This is the way you've always wanted to live.

Today's Action Plan: I will be in charge of my own right-eating plan. When I need nutritional help, I will get it.

October 30

Weight Slaves

*When I weighed 239 pounds, I thought I had no right to
be seen on the street, to eat in a restaurant, to live!*
Woman at Weight Watchers

You are a person with all the rights to live that other
people have. Your weight, whatever it is, doesn't change
that basic fact. You must accept this truth, or you can't
believe anything. You do accept this fact, don't you?
That's good!

Carry yourself like a winner everywhere you go. Do
you say, "I don't know how"? If so, watch people, of all
sizes. You'll easily be able to separate life's winners from
the walking apologies. The apologists have their shoulders hunched under stiff necks. They look at the ground,
casting furtive glances, hoping no one will notice them.
Their carriage is a sign that reads, "Don't approach me,
I'm unlovable!" Conversely, winners walk with shoulders
back, heads high, eyes curious about the world. Their
confident bearing is a banner which declares: "I'm a
beautiful person, you'd like to know me!"

Are you saying, "But it's so hard — there's a lot of
ridicule out there if you're overweight"?

Many people in this world have been ridiculed, ostra-
cized, and laughed at. Winners reject rejection because
they believe in their rights as humans. There's only one
right you don't have, the right to quit, to retreat into
apathy and self-pity. You won't let that happen, will
you? You bet you won't!

What have you done right today? You determined to
carry yourself like a winner. You rejected weight-slavery.

**Today's Action Plan: I will carry a sign that says, "I'm
a beautiful human being." I will never give up my rights.**

303

October 31

Get Out There and Live!

*He that resolves upon any great and good end has, by
that very resolution, scaled the chief barrier to it.*
Tryon Edwards

Let's say you're applying for work you really want —
the job of losing weight and changing your life. Now
make a mental resumé listing your qualifications for this
job. You wouldn't begin by berating yourself. You
wouldn't say, "I'm a stupid, rotten person who can't
even control food." Would you (as employer) want to
hire someone with qualifications like that? Of course not.

Clean up your personal resumé. If you wrote any
negative statements like the one above, delete them.
They disqualify you for the success you seek. Concentrate instead on your positive ideas and get into Action.

Get out there and live. You live in a fascinating world.
There are things you haven't done, people you haven't
met. There is beauty to enjoy. There are songs to sing,
great ideas to be learned.

You are a person who feels deeply. This makes you
uniquely capable of getting the most out of new experiences, moments of beauty and triumph. The world will
make way for people like you. But first, you must
become the person you want to be. There are three steps
to the open door: right-eating, exercise, and a self-
accepting view of yourself. One, two, three — go! Say
YES today, won't you?

What have you done right today? You decided to
clean out all the negative garbage from your "life
resumé."

Today's Action Plan: I will not disqualify myself for
the "job" of living thin. I will take steps to get out into
the world and live.

November 1

For the Health of It

Lethargy does not make fat; fat makes lethargy.
Source unknown

Are fat people lazy? A most pervasive stereotype of an overweight person is one who goes to any lengths to avoid physical exertion. There's even a joke in tennis that hefty players "have the longest arms." Frankly, these observations are unfair. Sedentary people don't always gain weight. But overweights are most always sedentary. There are two reasons. First, we tend to disown our bodies, focusing on activities that require the least physical commitment. Second, we avoid the embarrassment and harassment we might encounter if we exercise in public. But we pay a high price for physical unfitness, don't we?

Without a commitment to exercise you must eat less and less to maintain weight loss, thus jeopardizing good nutrition. And without exercise you don't get all those lovely pluses, like reduced appetite, increased weight loss, a sense of emotional well-being, better muscle and skin tone. But most of all, you won't get the sense of owning your own body.

Few people give regular exercise the six to eight weeks it takes to experience real changes. You are one of the few. Believe that, won't you, and give yourself time?

What have you done right today? You faced the difficulties of exercise for overweights. But you want the benefits, so you made a commitment to exercise today. That makes you someone special!

Today's Action Plan: I will give myself time to achieve body changes. I will see that looking and feeling great was worth the risk.

November 2

Junk Thinking

I wouldn't join a club that would have me for a member.
Groucho Marx

Most overweights feel they aren't worth the effort it takes to lose weight. That's why so many diets ultimately fail, and those who lose weight regain it. Then they push away others' affection, further devastating their self-image and possibility for success. They think, as in Groucho's classic joke, "If people love me, they must be losers." That's an example of junk thinking, isn't it?

But look at you! You took the self-hate out of weight loss. You learned the benefits of problem-solving. From this book you learned that your feelings are only a starting point. Emotional awareness is a game of feelings that satisfies briefly but doesn't help you make lifelong changes. In the end, discovering a feeling means nothing unless it's followed by commitment. Only time and plain hard work bring about change. This is the point at which most people fall down, but not you.

You've been learning Action skills. Use them to put more self-esteem into your self-image. Don't wait for the spirit to move you; take Action, dig in, and you move the spirit! Get the Action habit and soon you'll be shouting, "If they love me, they must be winners." Just try it and see, won't you?

What have you done right today? You learned that rejecting others because you thought yourself unworthy was junk thinking.

Today's Action Plan: I will remember that I am worthy of good things. I will use my Action skills today.

Create a Commercial

The grand essentials to happiness in this life are some-
thing to do, something to love,
and something to hope for.

Joseph Addison

You must come to realize that you are absolutely unique — your billions of cells are put together as none have been before and none will be again. One way you can illustrate this idea to yourself is to make a commercial. That's right, an advertisement like the ones you see on television. Sure it's a gimmick, but what have you got to lose except a bad self-image?

To build self-confidence, particularly before facing a tough prospect, top salespeople often recite short personal commercials. The theme is usually an "I look good, I feel fine" message. Sometimes it's designed to solve a special problem, like shyness or stammering.

Your own special commercial can go something like this:

As long as there's a (your name), there's Action, Reliability and Excellence. Use (your name) for the best right-eating, physical fitness, and a winning view of life. You'll receive all this, and big savings too. No weekly binges, no Monday morning martyrdom, no day-after depression. To top it off, you get 24-hour delivery, 365 days a year — at no extra charge. Buy (your name) today!

Use this commercial, or better yet, make your own. Learn it, and repeat it, when you're facing a tough day, won't you?

What have you done right today? You created your own commercial, a pep-talk for extra confidence.

Today's Action Plan: I will use my commercial when I need a mental boost. I will buy my own product — me.

The Shape of Things to Come

*If one only wished to be happy, this could be easily
accomplished; but we wish to be happier than other
people, and this is always difficult, for we believe others
to be happier than they are.*

Montesquieu

If you idealize thin people, think again. Their lives aren't
always models of satisfaction and excitement. True, they
usually don't have our health and social problems, but
being thin will not banish all human problems. You will
still deal with those when you reach your natural weight,
won't you?

Some overeaters feel cheated when they lose weight
and find their lives aren't fairy-tale perfect. There is
always give-and-take in personal relationships at home
and at work, no matter what your weight is. And
compliments and extra support fade when you reach
your goal weight. Suddenly others expect you to handle
problems without turning to food, just like everyone
else.

Your early weight-maintenance program can be a
disillusioning time because of your own unrealistic expectations. One woman said, only half-joking, "I thought
when I was thin I'd be able to play the piano without
taking lessons."

When you are thinner, you may not be more talented
or richer, but you will have a more attractive, energetic
body to live in, a new LifeWay that shows you how to
aim at goals and win. That's not a bad way to start your
thin life, is it?

What have you done right today? You took a realistic
look at thinness and decided it was worth the trip.

**Today's Action Plan: I will prepare myself by under-
standing that a thinner me won't be problem-free. I will
be a more understanding person for having been overweight.**

November 5

The Sunshine-maker

The person who can laugh with life has developed deep roots with confidence and faith — faith in oneself, in people and in the world, as contrasted to negative ideas with distrust and discouragement.

Democritus

The sixth Action MindStep tells you: **Make your own sunlight.** This may seem a trivial concept compared to the take-charge-of-your-life thrust of the other eleven MindSteps. But look again, won't you?

We overweights have our problems. In fact, we seem to have more than our share of burdens. We need laughter, don't we? Learning to relax and laugh is a link with the good life.

Laughter demolishes anger. That's why sometimes we resist laughing in the midst of upset; self-righteously we want to hang onto the drama a bit longer.

Laughter doesn't land on our doorstep. We must create it ourselves from our hope and determination to make our lives work better. Leave time for fun and laughter. Be a sunshine-maker, and every good laugh will be a mini-vacation in the midst of your day. Won't you like that?

What have you done right today? You took charge. You smiled, and laughed with a winner's gusto.

Today's Action Plan: I will let go of burdens and embrace laughter often today. I will make joy that does not depend on others.

Be Yourself

The most exhausting thing in life is being insincere.
Anne Lindbergh

Not being who you really are is a tragedy. You have talent, ambition, strength, and you've proved you're a fighter. But how do you reach the point where you become who you really are?

As much as possible, remove yourself from diet talk. All the what-I-ate-yesterday histories (OA members call them "foodalogs") tend to define you as only a food machine.

Lead a well-rounded life. Eating is not the only aspect of your life. High achievers have a variety of interests and relationships. They pay attention to their spiritual and emotional growth, too. Remember always that you are a person, not a size.

Seek direction rather than perfection. Your weight on a specific calendar day is less important than the direction you're going. Is your weight going down or has it stabilized? Do you feel great? These are results you want.

Compete with yourself, not others. True champions enjoy improving their own performance more than beating their competitors. One definition of a winner is someone who isn't self-defeating.

This is not just try-harder advice. If you choose, you have the power to improve the quality of your life. That's the point and that's what you want, isn't it?

What have you done right today? You decided not to seek perfection and to stop food-talk. You chose to lead a well-rounded life, to seek direction, and to compete only with yourself.

Today's Action Plan: I will be who I am, not what I think others expect. I will practice a winner's skills.

Are You Eating Too Much Fat?

It almost seems as if there's a conspiracy to keep our fat intake excessive.

Carol Flinders

Processed food, restaurant cooking, and most snack foods are usually far too high in saturated fats. You should do your own cooking as much as possible so you'll know how much fat you're eating. The diet most of us follow, even thin people, is 40 percent fat. This is a priority problem for you since your weight-loss eating plan should have less than 30 percent fat. Your right-eating plan pays attention to fat intake, doesn't it?

To keep your eating plan's fat content under 30 percent, you may consume only four to six tablespoons of fat a day.

Remember that a gram of fat has nine calories. So how do you pick a safe product? Read the label. If the food item has twelve grams (108 calories) of fat in a total of 400 calories, then it's 25 percent fat — right for your eating plan. On the other hand, based on the same measurement, you'll find that mayonnaise contains about 90 percent fat — definitely not recommended for your eating plan.

It takes a little extra time, but you want to take control of the fat in your food. When you do, you'll enjoy better health and appearance. That's what you want, isn't it?

What have you done right today? You learned a simple way to measure the fat in the food products you buy. It's part of the intelligent way you're taking charge of the food in your life.

Today's Action Plan: I will reduce the fat content of my food to 30 percent or less. I will concentrate on foods in this range.

November 8

A Fast-acting Cure for the Blues

Knowledge is not power. Action, which is knowledge in motion, does the work of the world.
Walter A. Heiby

A battle between mind and body can cause grief. When you know you need to eat less for weight loss but you continue to overeat and gain weight, you endure incredible turmoil. Depression and unhappiness are sure to follow. You know about that, don't you?

Today, return to a simple idea. Think, "I will act out my desire for a new LifeWay." With such a philosophy, conflict is removed, depression is banished. It is that simple.

As long as you are back to basics today, make a YES decision to "get more things going" in other areas of your life. It takes only a few minutes to make a right-eating decision for today. After that move away from preoccupation with food.

Stretch. Stimulate your mind. Associate with people who have new ideas. Grow in your job and social life.

The whole point of your new LifeWay is not merely to exchange an eating machine for a dieting machine. You've got more important things to do, better places to go, successes to achieve. The rest of your life beckons you on. Step smartly, won't you?

What have you done right today? You saw that the fastest cure for depression is erasing the conflict between what you want for your life and what you are actually doing. That is something important to remember from now on.

Today's Action Plan: I will act upon my desire for a new LifeWay. I will become part of the big world outside of my weight problem.

November 9

Reject Unfairness and Seek Support

All the art of living lies in a fine mingling of letting go and holding on.

Havelock Ellis

Some oaf laughs at you while you're taking a brisk walk in your neighborhood. A meddlesome nurse berates you because your weight goal doesn't correspond with her charts. A jealous acquaintance demeans your success. Such slights aren't fair, are they? Don't expect continual fairness. Unfair things happened to you before and may happen again. But it's not because you deserve to be treated cruelly. Reject unfairness without demeaning yourself. Do that, won't you?

Unfair people are selfish, emotionally immature, and confused. They're not right. They've got bigger problems than you do, unless you make their problems yours. And you do that if you carry around their image of you, rather than your own.

If you reject their unfairness, they lose, you win.

Now begin to seek and accept the good, kind, supportive people you know. Let go of the idea that fat makes you unworthy of love and acceptance. Hold on to what you are becoming through your right-eating, energizing, MindStepping LifeWay. You owe yourself this, don't you?

What have you done right today? You learned that people are often unfair, but it's their problem. You refuse to make their problem your problem. That's an excellent move.

Today's Action Plan: I reject the unfairness of others. I will win no matter what others say or do.

November 10

Think on these Things

*We think too small — like the frog at the bottom of the
well. He thinks the sky is only as big as the top of the
well. If he surfaced, he would have
an entirely different view.*

Mao Tse-Tung

There are five major themes running through this book.
You're probably aware of them, but as a strong support
for your new LifeWay you need to know them well.
Don't you think this would help?

1. Your conflict and unhappiness decrease in direct
   proportion to the harmony you achieve
   between your intent and Action.
2. You are capable as you are and have everything
   you need to become a winner.
3. Action creates motivations, not the other way
   around.
4. Action is a pre-condition for increasing your
   self-esteem.
5. You make your own choices. Others have power over you only if you choose to grant it.

Repeat these powerful themes. Learn them and use
them every day when the going gets tough. They'll keep
you strong. You want that, don't you?

What have you done right today? You "see the whole
sky." You are committed to applying the themes of this
book to your LifeWay.

Today's Action Plan: I will learn these power-filled
themes. When the going gets tough, I will use them for
strength.

November 11

Exercise for the Person Too Busy to Exercise

After my husband's heart attack, the doctor prescribed two miles of brisk walking to prevent another attack. If walking is that good for him, I figured it would be great for me.

Diet center speaker

You're a busy person and this is a fast-moving world. You say you don't have time to exercise in any regular way. Not so. Walking is the perfect exercise for people too busy to exercise. It fits into small time periods, and unlike running, swimming, or tennis, it needs no special clothes or places or even showering afterwards. Have you considered how easily you could fit walking into your busy day?

Stride ahead. Walking's natural rhythm has a relaxing quality, and at the same time it tones your body muscles, expands your lung capacity, helps weight loss, reduces fatigue, and makes you feel younger.

Walk every chance you get — to and from work or shopping, if that's possible. If not, take a walk break during your lunch hour.

Roughly fifteen average city blocks equal a mile. A slow pace will cover this distance in twenty minutes, a brisk pace will make it in thirteen minutes. Start slow and work up to brisk. Promenade today, won't you?

What have you done right today? You learned about an exercise that fits neatly into any busy schedule. You are determined to energize your body.

Today's Action Plan: I will walk whenever I get a few minutes. I will get many benefits from this most convenient form of exercise.

November 12

Your Margin of Tranquility

Without a certain margin of tranquility,
truth succumbs.

Ortega y Gasset

When you were overeating did you deliberately remove pleasure from your life? Did you say, "If I'm fat, I don't deserve to have fun?"

Now that you took charge of your overeating, energized your body, and adopted a positive view, you have begun to create an emotional comfort zone around your life.

Avoid being in a frantic rush. You don't have to hurry to lose weight, hurry to meet the right mate, hurry to have fun. Pleasure needn't be something you rush so frantically for that you miss the pleasure of this moment.

Live all the days of your life. Begin with today. Relax. Take time for meaningful ritual, a walk in the park, reading fine literature, or developing your inner spiritual life. Slow your frantic pace, and experience the beauty around you.

Isn't it wonderful to inject some tranquility into your life? But don't think of tranquility as only a passive, dreamy state. If based on the Action MindSteps, tranquility can be dynamic. Believe that, won't you?

What have you done right today? You put pleasure back into your life. You created an emotional comfort zone of right-eating and right-thinking.

Today's Action Plan: I will put pleasure into this day. I will add tranquility to my emotional life.

Keep Delivering

A fellow doesn't last long on what he has done. He's got to keep delivering as he goes along.
Carl Hubbell

Motivation — call it energy, drive, desire, or what you will — pervades psychology's literature. Years of studies about motivation have concluded that flashy, initial success doesn't always predict long-term performance. The most reliable predictor of success is commitment. You can see how that would be, can't you?

Commitment is a fire fueled by persistence. You develop a burning passion to pursue your goal and continually feed the flame of self-confidence with small, interim goals along the way.

Achievement-oriented people never stagnate. They learn constantly, adding to their knowledge every day. Ask yourself: What do I want to learn today? When you begin your day with such a goal, you won't dissipate time and energy in aimless activity.

Look around and see all the things you have yet to learn, things that will make a difference in your life. Learn about nutrition, about your own body and mind, and about the beautiful world you live in. When you do, you will keep moving toward your goals. This is your life's real work, isn't it?

What have you done right today? You realized that the most powerful thing you could give your life is commitment to the living goals you set for yourself.

Today's Action Plan: I will renew my commitment to the winning life. I will keep on delivering that commitment every day.

The Nature of Food Addiction

Facing a task of this magnitude (losing weight) requires fortitude, dedication and motivation. The patient must not be made to feel like a glutton or sinner.
The Merck Manual of Diagnosis and Therapy

You probably weren't born overweight, and you might not have been overweight as a child or adolescent. But sometime in your life you changed from eating-to-live to living-to-eat. When do you think that happened?

The change probably began when you first overate to help deal with stress. Soon your binges became less casual, more frequent, and planned. Eventually you overate when you felt good *or* bad.

As overeating increased you felt you needed larger portions or certain high-calorie foods. Food became a payoff for enduring frustrations and coping with daily stress. Finally, you no longer linked eating with pleasure or pain. All emotions caused cravings until cravings overwhelmed feelings.

Therefore, to control your overeating you must sever your emotional bond to food and make new emotional connections to success, to your body, and to your attitudes.

You've come so far. You've learned so much. You've found new ideas, new combinations of old ideas, unexpected thoughts, and more courage to go on. That's true, isn't it?

What have you done right today? You discovered the nature of an overeater's addiction. You know that what you once learned about food can be relearned.

Today's Action Plan: I will build new emotional connections omitting food. I will have courage to go on.

The Loneliness of a Long-time Overeater

Loneliness is the fear of love.

Ira Tanner

Many people are a little more alone than they once were. We move around so much, live in impersonal big cities or behind suburbia's fences. We leave families and childhood friends to move hundreds of miles away. We may even form more than one family in a lifetime. But being alone is not the same as loneliness. Lonely people feel disconnected from others and even from themselves. Have you ever felt the loneliness of having no one to turn to?

When you overeat you are lonely in a special way. You feel your loneliness inside, but what's worse, you believe you deserve to be lonely. You think, "I don't blame people for not liking me; after all, I'm pretty worthless."

You are self-conscious when you walk into a room full of people. You focus on your own feelings, reading negativity into other people's minds. It's difficult to project an open-for-friendship attitude when you are so self-focused. It's nearly impossible to start a friendship unless you consider the feelings of others as well as your own.

If you stick to it, your new LifeWay gives you confidence and increased self-esteem. You will begin to do wonderful things. Your MindStep attitudes will start to show. They're very attractive. Did you know that?

What have you done right today? You decided not to be lonely in a crowd. You plan to project an open-for-friendship attitude.

Today's Action Plan: I will be a friend to myself so that I can be a friend to others. I will believe that others are lucky to have me for a friend.

November 16

Your Working Dream

*Our destiny changes with our thought; we shall become
what we wish to become, do what we wish to do, when
our habitual thought corresponds with our desire.*
Orison Swett Marden

We see an endless stream of drastic diet regimens —
eating one fruit, taking one powder, drinking one liquid.
Presumably, these nutritional monstrosities are based on
the idea that overeaters love to punish themselves.
Medicine offers a flow of equally drastic remedies such
as bypass operations, jaw-wiring, and stomach-stapling.
These methods don't attempt to deal with overeaters'
minds. They do not take into account that "thinning" is
a process of the mind as much as the body. That's true,
isn't it?

Most of these panaceas insult overeaters by treating
them as passive objects for manipulation, rather than
active participants in their own recovery. The idea that
you have the ability and the right to take charge of your
life, to become a self-manager, may be discounted or
ignored.

Through the Twelve Action MindSteps you have
made your mind a powerful resource for changing your
body. It is natural that you want to follow your own
commands for living. Thus you have become focused on
your dream of a natural LifeWay. Even more important,
because of the principles of Action, you make your
dream a *working* dream. Isn't that right?

What have you done right today? You saw that you
have more power over your life than ever before.

**Today's Action Plan: I will become a self-manager. I
will be an active participant in my recovery from
overeating.**

Your Mind Matters

The used key is always bright.
Benjamin Franklin

Thoughts are real and powerful. Look at what you've accomplished through the power of thought. You have become what you are with the strength of your mind. Isn't that true?

The idea that the mind controls behavior doesn't imply that you, personally, can control everything that happens to you. But it does say that you have control over your own thoughts, and you control what you do about them. It means that when you confront a problem, you are in charge of how you deal with it. Most important, it means that your mind can control your overeating problem.

When you apply mind-solutions to your problem, you are authorizing yourself to create a control for overeating. Such creative thinking begins with giving yourself permission to work from the inside out, not from the outside in.

In the past you did not control overeating because of what others thought or said, and you weren't helped by the jobs or loves you lost, nor by circumstances that dictated that you should lose weight. None of these negative outside controls worked.

Today you know that your thoughts are what will change the circumstances of your life. The decision to take charge of the food in your life is a tangible event you made happen. Think of that, won't you?

What have you done right today? You saw how "mind over food" is the bright key to a thinner future.

Today's Action Plan: I will connect my creative mind to my overeating problem. I will become what my own thoughts direct me to be.

Whipping the Electric-egg-whisk Society

Since the early 1900s Americans have actually decreased their food intake, become more sedentary, and grown fatter. It's clear that the problem is not eating too much, but exercising too little.

Dr. Peter Wood

Great-grandmother fed the chickens, made two trips to the root cellar, pumped well water for washday, and fixed breakfast for ten — all before 8 a.m. Great-grandfather chopped wood, brought in the cows from pasture, milked and fed them — all before breakfast. What would they think of a society that found it necessary to invent the electric egg whisk? What do you think?

For years, overweight has been charged to gluttony. Of course overeating occurs. But it is erroneous to ignore the major contributor to contemporary overweight, lack of exercise.

Perhaps in the past, you viewed exercise as drudgery. Try a few new twists: vary your physical activity, think of exercise as play. You know, it takes very little exercise to do yourself good, and so little extra food to do yourself harm. A banana a day (72 calories) adds up to nearly an 8-pound-per-year weight gain. On the other hand, a minimum exercise program (walking a half-hour each day) shows up as a 20-pound-per-year weight loss.

Say no to food you don't need and YES to exercise. And while you're about it, throw away your electric egg whisk, won't you?

What have you done right today? You decided to get on the weight-losing track by exercising and following your food plan each day.

Today's Action Plan: I will discard electric-egg-whisk thinking. I will vary my energizing exercises for the fun of it.

November 19

Expect Victory

*Lack of faith in yourself, in what life will do for you,
cuts you off from the good things of the world. Expect
victory and you make victory.*

Preston Bradley

"Believe in yourself" isn't just a bumper-sticker phrase.
It's a practical tool. For example, the underdog Notre
Dame basketball team had to face undefeated UCLA, a
team which had amassed the longest winning streak in
basketball history. On the day before the big game,
instead of jittery exhortations to his players, the Notre
Dame coach gave his team a special drill. He had them
practice cutting the string basket off the hoop — a
victory ritual. To everyone's surprise (except the coach's)
Notre Dame won the contest by one point and the
champions climbed up to snip away the net and march
off the court, just as they had rehearsed. That's a grand
example of the power of belief, isn't it?

Expect victory. Practice success. Plan to win.

Having faith in your success doesn't mean you sit back
and wait for somebody to hand it to you. To ensure
victory, you have to plant yourself firmly in front of
destiny. Prepare yourself for victory with right-eating,
energizing your body, and winning attitudes.

A person with a winning attitude presumes victory.
Prepare to play on the winning team. "I will win" is the
most powerful positive I-gram you can send yourself.
Expect victory today, won't you?

What have you done right today? You adopted an
expectation of victory and worked to prepare yourself to
receive success.

**Today's Action Plan: I will prepare to win. I will
expect victory and accept nothing less.**

Planners Succeed

Success is planned for and planners have success.
                                        Larry Worman

Overeating brings chaos. Despite this, we tend to shy
away from putting structure into our lives. Perhaps
structure looks like too much trouble, so we procrastinate. How sad! There may be trouble in your life, but this
life, though imperfect, is the only one you have. Enjoy
it. With structure instead of chaos, you begin to realize
just how beautiful life can be. Will you think that way
for a moment?

Now spend a few minutes planning for success. If
you've read more than a few pages of this book, you
know the formula: set goals, make a commitment, take
Action, keep motivating yourself.

Motivation comes from two places. Outside rewards
are one source, but the most lasting motivation comes
from the confidence that "I'm doing this because I want
to, not because I have to."

This certainty that you are worthy of your best efforts
puts you in control of your thinking — and of your
planning. Be a planner for success and you will not fail.
Believe that, won't you?

What have you done right today? You planned for
success because this is the only life you have and you
want to make it a beautiful one.

Today's Action Plan: I will not postpone plans for my
life. I will plan because I want to do it, not because I
have to do it.

Worry Is Not Responsibility

Worry is a thin stream of fear trickling through the mind. If encouraged, it cuts a channel into which all other thoughts are drained.

Arthur Somers Roche

Some overeaters feel that if you worry a lot over your problem, it shows that you're doing something about it. There's a story about a man who constantly worried about elephants. He was so worried about being trampled that he burned incense to keep them away. "Nonsense," said a friend, "there are absolutely no wild elephants in this country." Replied the worrier, "See? My incense is working."

But alas for overeaters, worrying about the specter of eating doesn't work. Rather than warding off the problem, worry actually gives it life. For example, when you worry about overeating instead of taking positive Action, you think negative thoughts, pushing out positive ones and setting yourself up for failure. If instead of worrying, you use your energy to support your chosen LifeWay, success is far more likely. Can you accept this truth?

Worry takes valuable time. It keeps you so busy you don't have time to take Action on your real problems. Worry is a clever device your inner negative critic uses to keep you inactive. Become an active planner for a positive future, and you'll feel more in control. Your critic can't manage an optimist like you. That's true, isn't it?

What have you done right today? You decided to worry less about elephants and take Action on your real problems.

Today's Action Plan: I will stamp out worry with Action planning. I will decide what I want to change, and then do it, instead of just worrying about it.

November 22

No One Is Born to Fail

*The whole philosophy of failure can be summed up in
. . . three words, "What's the use?"*

Anonymous

One of the greatest moments in your life will come when
you realize that you're as good as anyone. Following
that revelation you will be open to this idea: you weren't
born to fail; you were born to succeed. On that morning
you'll have a feeling of wholeness and identity. Best of
all, you'll gain a sense of continuity with yourself that
you can depend on for life. From that moment on, you
will be good company for yourself. If that day hasn't
happened to you yet, it will soon. Believe that, won't
you?

Hasten that day by practicing "I am" rather than "I'm
not" attitudes. Say, "I am smart," "I am strong," and "I
am in control." This outlook will help you to see the
person you really are.

Get in the habit of being a can-do, not a can't-do
person. Winners are people who take charge, who let
nothing negative interfere with their plans. Taking
charge of their lives then becomes a series of right
Actions, no matter what. To winners, "What's the use?"
is a defeatist phrase which has no place in their vocabulary.

You belong to the Action people, to the winner's
circle. You were born to win. Isn't that right?

What have you done right today? You began working
for the greatest day of your life — the day when you'll
know that you are whole. You became an "I am" person.

**Today's Action Plan: I will be a winner. I will never
ask, "What's the use?"**

November 23

Exercise Like a Winner

*Overzealous beginners start out too quickly
and intensely with their program, and wind up
burning out mentally or else placing
too much stress on not-yet-well-developed muscles.*
Dr. Jesse DeLee

We all-or-nothing people are apt to start an exercise
program too fast, go too far, and become disillusioned
about exercise. The key to exercise benefits is to find an
activity or sport you enjoy and then progress from easy
to more difficult, isn't it?

It is particularly important that overweights take it
slow but steady. If you want to run, start walking, move
to a jog, and then to running. If you find running too
hard on feet or joints, then pull back to a jog or even a
"wog" — a walk-jog. You'll get just as much or more
weight-loss benefit, because without injuries you'll be
able to stick to it.

It's never too late in life to aim for total fitness. This
may be tough on those of us who are overweight,
because we've got weight to lose as well as conditioning
to achieve, but we can be winners, too. (Ever thought of
yourself as a jock?)

Outside the realm of physical well-being, there's a
benefit to exercise that's never mentioned: it helps give
your life structure. When you program exercise into your
day, your other activities must be better organized to
make them all fit.

Start slow, build your time and skill, pull back when
necessary — but keep at it. There's a winning jock in
you, isn't there?

What have you done right today? You subscribed to
the old proverb: Slow and steady wins the race.

**Today's Action Plan: I will aim for total fitness. I will
exercise like a winner.**

The Pain of Knowing

Unless there be correct thought, there cannot be any action, and when there is correct thought, right action will follow.

Henry George

Working with the MindSteps every day means we deal with realities. This pursuit leads to discovering a great potential within ourselves — the capacity to take charge of our thoughts, bodies, and affairs. But this knowledge also leads to a new (but treatable) pain, the pain of knowing we could have done much more than we've done. When there was no awareness of potential, when we thought we were limited, there was no point in striving. But now, as our capabilities open to us, knowing how much more we can do has to be dealt with. You've experienced this feeling, haven't you?

How do you deal with your new-found potential? Remember, as a child, when you begged to play a game with older children? Finally they gave in and let you try. You couldn't keep up, but you knew you *should* because others could. Did you work until you mastered the game, or did you walk out saying, "I don't like that dumb game anyway"?

You are in the process of becoming all that you can be. You will be greatly challenged. You can pronounce these challenges "dumb," and walk away. On the other hand, you can rise to the challenge and give the game of life the best you've got. That makes better sense, doesn't it?

What have you done right today? You learned that the pain of knowing is discovering the glorious potential that lies hidden inside you.

Today's Action Plan: I will play every game up to my potential. I will be in charge of my thoughts, body, and daily life.

Exercise Your Self-esteem

*You come into the world with nothing, and the purpose
of your life is to make something out of nothing.*
H. L. Mencken

You increase your chances for success by reading this
book each day. There probably isn't one idea on these
pages that you weren't already aware of on some level.
You might even have told yourself some of the same
things you read. However, you didn't follow your own
good advice. Seeing it here in print helps to crystallize
what you know is right for you, doesn't it?

Today when you promise yourself you're going to lose
weight, you'll follow through. Your new LifeWay won't
allow you to make a promise that you have no intention
of keeping. This would undermine your self-trust, and
you need all you've got.

Take the time today to complete one simple task you
are avoiding but know needs doing. This will increase
your self-esteem. (In the past, you never seemed to find
the right time to tackle tasks you didn't feel like doing.)

Suppose you fall down today. Don't focus all your
attention on the fall. You'll become too discouraged to
take a risk. Focus your attention on getting up and
beginning again.

Reinforcing your positive Actions puts you in a good
learning position, able to make something wonderful of
your life. Exercise your self-esteem today, won't you?

What have you done right today? You felt stronger
because you were reasonable with yourself. Nothing
overwhelmed you, and you were encouraged to reach
for your goals.

Today's Action Plan: I will listen to my own good
advice. I will exercise my self-esteem so that I will be
receptive to good ideas.

November 26

Exercise — a Natural Therapy

> *. . . tension is trapped energy.*
> Naura Hayden

Tension is a familiar feeling for most overeaters. We can thank tension-eating for a good many of our extra pounds. Relaxation therapy and hypnotism are recognized non-drug controls for tension. But a different way to manage tension is to treat it as trapped energy which we can release daily through physical exercise. That's an interesting thought, isn't it?

Whether tension is of the stiff-upper-lip or the screaming-meemie variety, imagine it as energy bursting to get out. Now think of play, movement, and exercise as energy safety valves allowing you to dissipate tension harmlessly while losing weight and toning your body at the same time.

It's miraculous! There are few things in this world with so many physical and mental benefits all wrapped up in a few minutes of daily commitment.

Get moving today. A half-hour walk is heaven compared to a half-hour food binge. Likewise your stationary bicycle is far better for you than a battle with your boss, mate, or neighbor.

Holding onto tension is part of a loser's mentality. Getting rid of it (and getting so many benefits too) is a smart winner's mentality. There it is. The choice is obvious, isn't it?

What have you done right today? You released your tension-energy the winning way, with exercise. Making smart choices is the reason you're a thinner winner.

Today's Action Plan: I will not overeat because of tension build-up. I will take my nerves out and exercise them.

November 27

Two Chairs

*...I think everyone's second business is their occupation
and that their first business is to know themselves.*
                                                    Jo Coudert

A strange inner struggle wages inside most overeaters.
One part of us is defiant and says, "Don't you dare
make me eat less, exercise more, and believe all those
silly take-charge principles." But the other part shouts,
"Help! Somebody, *please*, help me stop!" How can both
these thoughts co-exist in one brain? You know the
answer — not very well. Isn't that right?

Play a mind game. Imagine two chairs facing each
other — your "help-me" self in one chair, your "defiant"
self seated opposite. Now let "defiant" scream how it
hates knuckling under to authority. Next have "help me"
explain how fighting structure and rules has always
gotten you in trouble, how unhappy you are with
overeating, and about your decision to change all that.
"Defiant" may argue, make demands, and stamp its feet,
but will offer no alternative to overeating.

Sometimes it helps to sort out problems with such
role-playing. Doing so can be an effective way to
demonstrate how determined you are to follow your new
LifeWay; to show yourself that you won't let anyone,
even your own defiant self, get in your way. That's
wonderful, isn't it?

What have you done right today? You played a mind
game that helped you sort out what you really want.

**Today's Action Plan: I will not overeat because of my
old childish defiance of authority. I will make it my
business to know myself.**

The Love of Your Life

When you know who you are and you realize what you can do, you can do things better at forty than when you're twenty.

Shirley MacLaine

Isn't it sad when adults think of themselves as deprived children, unloved and unlovable? This is not just a way to evoke sympathy, but a real gut feeling for many overeaters. What can be done to erase such a negative outlook?

You have to *feel* loved. It's not that most unhappy people aren't lovable, they feel unloved.

To feel lovable, acknowledge the loving things you do for others — the little services you normally ignore when you consider your lovability. Have you visited a sick person, fixed a child's hurt, listened sympathetically to a friend's troubles? All these are loving acts.

Make a mental list of the lovable qualities that you usually hide from others. Have you worked for or given to a charity, cared for a stray animal, written a letter of sympathy, laughed aloud, or sung joyously? All these are lovable qualities.

Just for today be a parent to yourself. Give yourself loving attention and praise for all the kind, thoughtful, generous gifts you give to others, and accept the love and attention offered by the people who love you. It's about time you had some recognition. Do it, won't you? Say YES.

What have you done right today? You forced yourself to face the loving and lovable parts of yourself.

Today's Action Plan: I will nurture myself. I will accept my loving and lovable qualities so that I will allow myself the happiness of food control.

November 29

Your Verbal Diary

It is the disease of not listening, the malady of not marking, that I am troubled withal.
William Shakespeare

Do you hide your emotions from others? Even from yourself? Sometimes we think this keeps us safe, but it endangers us more than we know. To keep those feelings locked inside, we have regularly smothered them with food. Express your feelings, won't you?

Sometimes we recognize this need, but we don't know how to act on it. Here's a way to learn what you're feeling and how to express it:

For the next week, set aside fifteen minutes at the end of each day. Tape-record your thoughts and feelings about the day's events. If you have no recorder, write them down for reading aloud.

At the end of the week, play back your tape (or recite your written diary) and listen, really hear, what you've said to yourself. Pay attention to what you felt and how you expressed those feelings. Now, how many of these feelings are so dreadful they couldn't be shared with someone dear to you? Not many. Pick two or three feelings (the ones you decide are appropriate) and express them to a sympathetic friend or relative. You learn to share feelings by sharing feelings. That's a simple solution to opening yourself to others.

Keeping a verbal diary can make a difference — pounds of difference, because stuffing feelings encourages you to stuff food. You're willing, aren't you?

What have you done right today? You saw how you held feelings inside of you by stuffing them down with food. You learned that sharing feelings is a better way to cope with them.

Today's Action Plan: I will start my verbal diary tonight. I will express my feelings so I won't have to smother them by overeating.

The Three R's of Friendship

What we see depends mainly on what we look for.
John Lubbock

Do you think you shouldn't burden your friends with your problems? If you do, you're ignoring a source of emotional support. Such friendly support doesn't just make life easier for you, it keeps your motivation high. And motivation is the life-blood of your right-eating, body energizing, and attitude-changing LifeWay. You can see how vital emotional support is to you, can't you?

Gain a friend's emotional support by following the Three R's:

1. Reaching out. Simply let your friends know that you need them.
2. Right person. Pick the right friend to share your emotional problem with, one who will be understanding.
3. Realistic expectations. Don't expect too much or too little from your friends; be realistic. A sympathetic ear is often quite enough.

When you share emotional problems with friends, you pay them the highest compliment. You show that you trust them and respect their judgment. You see that, don't you?

What have you done right today? You let go of any feelings of being a burden to your friends. You used the Three R's to gain the emotional support you need to win.

Today's Action Plan: I will reach out for emotional support when I need it. I will be willing to share my problems to safeguard my right-eating plan.

December 1

Where to Start and Stay

To live is to change, and to be perfect is to have changed often.
Cardinal Newman

If you've been overweight for some time, your weight probably is the central fact of your existence. It may limit your choice of work and your social roles and predetermine your attitudes about yourself. You may see yourself as an outcast, helpless, and hopeless. You may be caught in a vicious circle of low self-esteem and overeating. While most of the help you seek to break this circle addresses only the overeating problem, these pages also concentrate on combating low self-esteem. Thus, as you raise your feelings of self-worth, right-eating will be more natural for you. You see that, don't you?

You are a worthwhile, deserving person as you are. You are a valid person regardless of your present size. That is a simple fact.

But there is another fact. You live in a thin-oriented society. If you're overweight, that means you will probably live better as a thinner person, and enjoy improved health, looks, and energy. But basically you must choose between stepping into a real, if sometimes unfair, world, or living in a make-believe world of overeating. This is the choice you make every day, isn't it?

What have you done right today? You have decided to keep your self-esteem high and live comfortably in the real world.

Today's Action Plan: I will accept my personal value. I will make a choice each day to remove food as the center of my existence.

December 2

You Decide What Rules You'll Live With

*Man is not what he thinks he is, but what he thinks,
he is.*

Elbert Hubbard

Submerged defiance is a part of many overeaters' make-ups. It causes us to resist the kind of orderliness that right-eating, physical and mental fitness creates. You may think the structured way of life sounds too oppressive or too routine. Think again, won't you?

Did you know that, as an overeater, you abide by certain rules, too? It you think an Action MindStep day is restrictive, check the conditions overeaters impose on themselves:

1. Overweights should not buy nice clothes, disagree with friends, or believe compliments.
2. Overweights should never enjoy food, and always postpone living until they are thin.
3. Overweights don't deserve satisfying relationships with those of the other gender.
4. Overweights should never say "no" to the demands of others.
5. Above all, overweights should never praise themselves or feel good about anything they do.

Which set of rules will you follow, the overeater's rules or the Twelve Action MindSteps? It's a paradox, but the freedom to overeat carries with it the most restrictions, and your new Action MindStep way of living offers the most freedom. Choose freedom from overeating, won't you?

What have you done right today? You saw that the "rules of overeating" imposed the most restrictions on your life, the MindStep LifeWay the least.

Today's Action Plan: I will follow the plan that allows me maximum freedom. I will love freedom from overeating.

Do You Dislike Other Overweights?

There is very little difference in people, but that little difference makes a big difference. The little difference is attitude. The big difference is whether it is positive or negative.

W. Clement Stone

A woman boarded an airliner en route to a weight-losers convention. To her dismay, she was seated next to a man who was so obese that two seats and two belts had to be specially rigged to fit him. "I was so embarrassed," she recalled. "I didn't want others in the plane to identify me with this fat man. It took me a long time to undertand my feeling of loathing. Here I was, treating him as I had been treated myself. In a flash of insight, I knew that my animosity toward him was also directed at myself. Even though I had long felt the unfairness of society's attitude toward fat people, I had assimilated it and turned it against this man and myself." How would you honestly feel in this woman's place?

Some of us overweights have incorporated our society's disgust with fat, we look down on other fat people as deviants. We actually feel dislike for other overweights. This attitude is a disguised self-punishment.

When you have compassion for other overweights, you have compassion for yourself. You need more compassion to allow yourself to win, don't you?

What have you done right today? You took responsibility for your attitude. You had compassion for those who have not yet found their own way.

Today's Action Plan: I will have compassion for myself so that I can know compassion for others. I will not punish myself by assimilating society's disgust for fat, thereby making self-love impossible.

December 4

Five Favorite Fat Alibis

I like a state of continual becoming, with a goal in front and not behind.

George Bernard Shaw

Most of us who've had many diet setbacks had to find reasons for our failures. Do you recognize any of these?

1. "Mother forced me to eat when I was young."
2. "I cook for others, so I'm around food all day."
3. "I can't throw food out; my spouse calls it wasteful."
4. "Everyone in my family is fat."
5. "I'm so nervous, I can't stop eating."

The old excuse, "It's my glands," has been so thoroughly debunked, we don't use it anymore.

When you adopted the winning attitudes of the Twelve Action MindSteps, you assumed responsibility for your overeating and what it did to your body and life. That was necessary. We can't go back and change our childhood or our genes, and we can't force others to change. But we can change ourselves, create attainable goals, and adopt the strategies that will take us to them.

Often, as a final excuse, we throw up our hands and say, "I can't stand another diet!" This is doomsday thinking. Say instead: "I can't stand another day of overeating!" Now that's an idea you can stand forever, isn't it? Say YES.

What have you done right today? You let go of all excuses for postponing your life. You adopted winning MindStep attitudes with goals.

Today's Action Plan: I will reject excuses for failure. I will embrace self-responsibility for my overeating so that I can take Action.

December 5

You Can Help Yourself

Why let luck decide?

Gilbert Barnes

The whole idea of will power to solve weight problems has fallen on hard times. But if you translate will power into concepts such as self-reliance, strength of purpose, and faith in oneself, you can see that it can play a part in recovery. Today most alcoholics and other drug-users, smokers, and overeaters (lumped together as substance abusers) share the point of view that no one can kick an addiction alone. In most cases this is correct. But with strength of mind, you can add immeasurably to the help you get from support groups or from medical, psychological, and weight-loss professionals. Do you think that's possible?

Addiction is a mix of biological factors, but it is also determined by a person's attitudes and expectations. Most people biologically sensitive to substances can triumph over them — if they believe they can.

It may be an old-fashioned idea, but your own determination can change your life for the better. There is far more strength in you than you might think. Even if you need extra help to lick an addiction to overeating, others can't help you unless you give them your strength to build on. The point is that strong-minded people must believe, with everything they have, that they can do it. With that attitude recovery is not only possible, but inevitable. You believe that, don't you?

What have you done right today? You considered the possibility that determination, the power of your mind, and faith in yourself can help work miracles.

Today's Action Plan: I will use my strength of will, whatever my choice of methods. I will believe I can stop abusing food.

339

What's Good for the Body Is Good for the Mind

*The idea is to keep moving. Even a little bit is better
than none . . .*

Dr. Everett L. Smith

You've discovered something you didn't expect from
regular daily exercise, haven't you? When you exercise,
you can't help having a sunnier outlook on life. It is well
accepted that exercise increases endurance and muscle
strength and decreases your blood pressure and heart
rate. But people often are taken by surprise by the
pleasant mental and emotional side effects of exercise.
When you exercise you're clearly less depressed and
more hopeful, aren't you?

At least once today, do enough extra moving to make
your heart beat faster. You can do it by walking faster
than normal, by dancing, or by practicing a good
routine of calisthenics. The effects will last all day. Your
muscle cells will burn more fat — even if you take a nap
afterwards.

The best thing is that exercise will not make you
hungrier. Just the opposite. You'll want less to eat. How
many thousands of dollars have you spent on ways to
decrease your appetite? Here's one that costs nothing and
works better than any pill, potion, or magic diet on the
market.

Aren't you glad you're saving all that money while
losing all those pounds?

What have you done right today? You moved more
today and put more sunshine into your life — no matter
what the weather is like outside. You have something
that really works to reduce your appetite and weight. It's
a miracle!

Today's Action Plan: I will not resist the idea of
incorporating exercise into my life today. I will move
more and enjoy life more.

December 7

Your Greatest Discovery

*Putting off an easy thing makes it difficult; putting off a
hard one makes it impossible.*

George H. Lorimer

One day you will reflect that the most important
discovery of your life was the untapped power of your
own mind. You can read books, hear lectures, or collect
diplomas, but none of these scholarly pursuits can give
you more power to change your life than you already
possess. This is an exciting concept, isn't it?

Your power of thought rules your inner world. If you
declare, "I feel awful," you will be sick today. But if you
say, "I feel terrific — this will be another opportunity to
live fully!" then you will have empowered your day with
healthy optimism.

Today your mind rules your destiny, forms your
living environment, changes your personality. Today as
you think — negatively or positively — you harm or
heal yourself.

Perhaps you thought that eating-control comes as a
process of revelation — a flash of light, followed by
sudden power over food and personal peace. What if
you realized that you can make your own flash of light?
Think what freedom this gives you. Rather than being
helpless at the hands of unseen, uncontrollable forces,
you can make the necessary changes to meet the
demands of your day. It means you are totally capable,
doesn't it?

What have you done right today? You discovered the
power of your positive mind to change your destiny
from food-dependence to food control.

Today's Action Plan: I will use my thought power to
take charge of overeating. I will make my own flash of
light.

December 8

Your Perfect Right

Self-distrust is the cause of many of our failures.
Christian N. Bovee

Some overeaters have such a deep-seated distrust in themselves, they don't think they deserve the same rights as other people — thinner people. We become martyrs to our abundant flesh, unable to grant ourselves the slightest pleasure. This punishing and limiting attitude closes off pleasure, as well as potential solutions to our food problem. You see how important self-trust is, don't you?

You have rights, too:

> • You have a perfect right to deny unreasonable requests — graciously, but always firmly.
> • You have a perfect right to wear the colors and clothes styles you like and to walk in the sun without a navy blue coat to hide under.
> • You have a perfect right to exercise in public without harassment. (Anyone who says something derogatory is absolutely wrong, not you.)
> • You have a perfect right to use your talents at home, at work, or at a social gathering, no matter what you weigh.

Don't let your all-rightness depend on anything but what your MindStep attitudes tell you is your right. If you catch yourself saying, "I don't dare," or "I can't," send yourself a positive I-gram: "Yes, I can, and I have a perfect right to do so." Aren't you happy to be in control?

What have you done right today? You learned that you already have every right you need. Trust yourself.

Today's Action Plan: I will not be a martyr to my weight. I will use my rights.

December 9

Be Your Best Friend, Not Your Worst Enemy

Most people who engage in self-destructive behavior have simply chosen an ill-advised method of getting relief from the pain of their lives.

Dr. John W. Bush

Did you ever get angry at the fate that got you into the overeating mess? Whatever or whoever did it was your worst enemy. Can it be, though, that your worst enemy was you? Impossible, you say? It was very possible if you clung to overeating and it blocked your happiness. Using food to cope with a problem unrelated to physical hunger was self-defeating. Food binges solved no living problem, but created a new one — fat. That's true, isn't it?

There's a special gift for you on this page, the promise to show you a best friend.

Find a mirror. Right now, with this book in hand, get to the nearest mirror. Now look in it. The person you see — no, don't look away — that person is your best friend. Before you sit down again, take one Action to prove your friendship. No, no — don't make another future promise. *One Action is worth more than a thousand promises.*

Tell your mirror image, "Today, I will work the Action Plan at the bottom of this page. I will do it for you, no matter how hard it is." That sounds like a good friend talking, doesn't it?

What have you done right today? You decided to be your own best friend, not your worst enemy. You're somebody you'd like to know.

Today's Action Plan: Today I will follow my right-eating plan, exercise, and MindStep attitudes. I will send only positive I-grams to my best friend.

The Secret of Weight Maintenance

Exercise is the great appetite equalizer.

Anonymous

Regular physical activity helps you stabilize your weight. Of course, food portion control is important, but it's not the only solution, as once thought. The secret to maintaining your weight after shedding pounds is to continue your exercise program. If your scales show your weight is up, increase your exercise. You can agree so far, can't you?

When you arrive at your natural weight (that weight you've decided is most comfortable for you), you should give some thought to expanding your exercise repertoire. Check with your docter before starting, but consider skiing (especially the marvelously aerobic cross-country type), snowshoeing, racquetball, volleyball, or distance running.

Weight maintenance requires increased self-discipline, and exercise boosts self-discipline. Your mind becomes more focused, your thoughts concentrated, your energies channeled.

After exercising, you're in your own self-made world, physical energy spent, but mind clear and strengthened. Controlled eating then becomes just an extension of your physical and mental discipline. Have you experienced this yet?

What have you done right today? You saw you could stabilize your natural weight with exercise. You know that the whole gamut of exercise is now open to you.

Today's Action Plan: If my weight is above my natural level, I will exercise longer. I will look for new exercises to help maintain my weight goal.

December 11

The Special Person Inside You

*Don't bother just to be better than your contemporaries
or predecessors. Try to be better than yourself.*
William Faulkner

There is a special person inside you — a good, energetic,
achieving person — trying to get out. That person was
kept prisoner, condemned to unhappiness as long as you
indulged in anger, guilt, and self-ridicule. Tragically,
some of us almost destroy that special person before we
find our way. Have you met that special person you are?

You have the ability to think yourself through your
overeating and living problems. You don't need special
equipment; your miracle-working mind and your positive new LifeWay are enough to do the job.

There are few guarantees except this: while you search
for the special you, you grow; and as you grow, your
life changes for the better.

You are qualified to help yourself. Channel all the
anger, guilt, and self-ridicule into constructive Action.
Draw upon your positive self-image, your confidence,
your beliefs, and your accomplishments — show them,
share them. It will soon be clear that the special person
inside you has come out. Do it today, won't you? Say
YES.

What have you done right today? You looked inside
yourself and found a special person, one that is good,
energetic, and achieving. You freed that person.

Today's Action Plan: I will take the MindStep Life-
Way so that I can become who I really am. I will bring
out my best.

You're Not Alone

To feel that one has a place in life solves half the
problem of contentment.

George E. Woodberry

When you slip — go off your eating plan — you're not
alone. When you feel like a miserable failure, call
yourself unprintable names, you're not alone. When
your chin is on the ground and you're ready to give up
on the whole world for good, you're not alone. Many,
many others have felt that way too. Remember that,
won't you?

When you get down on life, on yourself, it's usually
because you've drifted away from your three basic,
simple needs: right-eating, exercise, and a winning attitude. You got too smart for all that basic stuff, and quit.
When you feel yourself getting in trouble, check to see
what you've decided you don't need to do any longer.
Then start doing it again.

Next, do two things. First, *talk* yourself out of a
slump. Winners talk out loud to themselves, tell themselves what they need to hear as no one else can.
Second, *work* yourself out of a slump. There is never a
substitute for taking Action; it is the great motivator, the
healer of problems. You understand, don't you?

What have you done right today? You have learned
that everyone slips — you aren't alone. You see that in
order to win, you have to get into Action each time you
stumble. Now you've got it!

Today's Action Plan: I will understand that others
have slipped too, that a slip can be part of my recovery.
I will get right up and continue.

December 13

The Success in Rejection

. . . few setbacks are as devastating as rejection . . .
Dr. David Burns

You phone a relative who is too busy to talk with you.
A coworker you admire takes a coffee break without
you. A sales clerk waits on a customer who arrives after
you. Everyone feels twinges of pain from such incidents.
But you may regard such acts as rejection and proof of
your unworthiness. What nonsense! Rejection is an idea,
an abstract one at that. You can't touch it and it can't
exist unless you permit it. Do you see?

The key to recovering from rejection (after you have
firmly disallowed it) is to use it as an occasion to
reaffirm your value. But that's not what most overeaters
do. Instead of affirming their self-worth, they sabotage
themselves. They see rejection as proof that they are
inept, unlovable, and unworthy of opportunity. "Why
try again?" they ask. The result is a pernicious circle of
blaming, inferiority, and low expectations.

Stop taking rejection so seriously, exaggerating it, and
beating yourself over the head with it. You rate love and
acceptance. Most of all, you deserve your own support.

Don't place your self-esteem on the line every time
you assume someone rejects you. Achieving success
means taking risks, and with risks, you may get some
rejection. So what? Remember, every rejection is merely
another chance to reaffirm yourself and thereby succeed.
Accept that, won't you?

What have you done right today? You learned that
you are the one who gives rejection its capacity to hurt.
Unless you assist it, it has no power of its own.

Today's Action Plan: I will not give life to a rejection
by agreeing with it. I will use rejection as a stepping
stone to success, as a winner should.

How Did It Feel to Be Fat?

It helps me to remember how miserable I was — the contrast is enough to make me want to maintain my weight loss.

Diet group speaker

Occasionally, recovering overeaters need to remember — even say out loud — the negative feelings they once held about themselves. Once those feelings were impossible to confront; now it is a great relief to speak of them in the past tense. You wouldn't trade one minute of your present LifeWay for a whole day of overeating, would you?

What's it like to be fat? It's not being able to cross your legs. It's hating words like plump, stout, chubby, and obese. It's being out of breath. It's buttons straining and thighs chafing. Remember?

That's not all. It's covering your stomach when sitting, always pulling at clothes. It's feeling bloated and ugly. It's always being embarrassed in public, never relaxed. Remember?

It's feeling ashamed, sick, guilty, and angry. It's not caring, because you feel you're worthless and beyond help, so you keep eating more than ever before. Remember?

Let these sad memories of overeating spur you to renewed MindStep Action. Let them ignite your plans for a thinner-winner way of life. Today you'll use negative memories to power positive Actions, won't you?

What have you done right today? You haven't forgotten the misery of overeating, and you are determined to make new and wonderful memories for yourself.

Today's Action Plan: I will remember the fat days so I know how far I've come. Today I will make thin memories.

December 15

Defeat Your Fat Denial Mechanisms

*One should . . . be able to see that things are hopeless
and yet be determined to make them otherwise.*
F. Scott Fitzgerald

Overeating created an underlying self-hate and shame,
which could only be appeased by more overeating. It
was a steel-jawed trap which you felt powerless to escape
from. Denial was the only way you could maintain a
shred of self-respect, so you concealed your weight with
loose clothing, you rationalized that everyone gained as
they aged, and you denied that you enjoyed sports or
dancing. If you couldn't drive someplace, you didn't go.
Clothes became larger and larger, breath shorter and
shorter. Finally, some trauma forced you to face yourself
and your denial mechanisms fell apart. Is your story
something like that?

Now is the best time to resolve never to let your fat
denial mechanisms work again. Refuse to see or use food
as a pacifier. Begin to see your life and your body as
your top priorities. Believe that you must take charge of
food if you want to do the things you denied yourself, if
you want to live a life of achievement, *if you want to
live at all.*

Make yourself the first priority in your life and you
will succeed. There's no other way. You see that, don't
you?

What have you done right today? You rejected fat
denial mechanisms that only served to delay really living
your life.

**Today's Action Plan: I will base my daily life on the
MindStep Action principles. I will never deny my top
priority again.**

December 16

Be an Inspiration

*An unexpected benefit of pain is the opportunity, even
the necessity, to be courageous.*

Anonymous

You can be an inspiration to your family, diet group,
and coworkers. As you lose weight, other overweights
(or even thins) will turn to you because they will see in
you attitudes they feel lacking in their own life. And
they will be right, won't they?

Your three-part LifeWay is a creative living process
which makes you fascinating to other people. Think
about it. In your recreation process you heal your inner
pain, restructure your self-image, and rebuild your body.
All this takes courage, and courage is inspiring. Inspiration is catching, infectious. The more you help other
people, the more firm your new attitudes will be.

So be a role model. But be aware of pitfalls. Don't let
your admirers put you on a pedestal, and don't begin to
think that your success removes you from temptation. It
doesn't. You must make your LifeWay a lifelong priority.

Your courage and your discipline will be a powerful
inspiration to other people. You will have succeeded at a
great task, a process others will want to copy. Help
them, won't you?

What have you done right today? You saw that you
can be a source of inspiration for other people. You will
help them, but you resolved to keep your own program
number one.

**Today's Action Plan: I will grow so that I can help
others. I will inspire others, while reinforcing my own
LifeWay.**

December 17

Command Therapy

The rhythm of life is intricate but orderly, tenacious but
fragile. To keep that in mind is to hold
the key to survival.

The Hon. Shirley M. Hufstedler

You need daily healing because few things are so stressful
as being overweight in a thin-is-in world. Controlling
stress and tension is essential to taking charge of your
health. Do you have a way to reduce stress and focus
your healing power?

To be your own best healer, take control of the
stresses in your life. Create a little inner refuge at
stressful times of day or places where you are prone to
overeat. Relax and remember a feeling of happiness, then
direct that feeling to the part of your body that needs it
most. If you feel hungry but know that you ate recently,
focus those happy, warm feelings on your stomach.
Your hungry feeling will fade.

You can go further yet with a technique called command therapy. Controlling your body is the principle
behind command therapy, which was originally designed
to aid cancer patients. For overweights, the method
requires that you imagine bad fat cells being hunted
down and devoured by good thin cells. Then imagine
yourself healing by visualizing yourself thin. Amazingly,
the technique has helped seriously ill people survive
beyond all expectations. Why can't this method help you
visualize your own body destroying the fat cells? It's
another way to take control of your body, isn't it?

What have you done right today? You will focus your
mind's healing powers on your weight problem.

Today's Action Plan: I will visualize thin cells attack-
ing and replacing fat cells. I will be in charge of my own
health.

December 18

Take Today — All the Way

I feel very happy to see the sun come up every day. I feel happy to be around. What I hope that my life's works will do is to declare a condition of joy. I like to take this day — any day — and go to town with it.
James Dickey

This is a new day, a new challenge, and it begins for you with your next heartbeat. Think about this. You have never lived this day before, never put your stamp on this day before. Never spoken, walked, laughed, or worked in this day. You're in charge of what you do with this day, aren't you?

Use this day efficiently; use all of it to further your goals. Sometimes we overeaters feel that we are victims of time. Time seems to work against us. Make time work for you today; allow it to become a self-valuing, productive experience. You need that! And you deserve it, too.

The first and greatest step today is to integrate all of your day into your right-eating, exercise, and Action MindStep program. Your LifeWay doesn't come second. It's never an afterthought; it's your first thought. It lights your way and prepares you for that "condition of joy" Dickey talked about. Think about that "condition of joy." You could take a day like that, couldn't you? Say YES.

What have you done right today? You saw that today is fresh, waiting for you to make it a triumph. And you will, too!

Today's Action Plan: I will make maximum use of today. I will integrate my three-part living program into the next twenty-four hours so that wonderful things become possible.

December 19

Rules of Self-esteem

The noble soul has reverence for itself.
Friedrich Nietzsche

Have you become an adult? No, it's not a silly question, because overeaters often treat themselves as bad children who need to be punished. When you treat yourself this way, you smother self-esteem, don't you?

Here are five ways you can start treating yourself as an adult:

1. Don't belittle yourself. Constant negative I-grams like, "I can't do anything right," are untrue and unkind.
2. Don't threaten yourself. "If you do that one more time . . . " thoughts destroy self-esteem. You may have to make the same mistake again before you learn.
3. Don't overprotect yourself. When you always remove yourself from risk, you see yourself as someone who can't handle mistakes. Your self-confidence is erased.
4. Don't play hopscotch with the MindSteps. When you train yourself to do something new, you must be consistent and systematic.
5. Don't use guilt as a motivator. "If I don't do that, I'm a rotten person" thoughts can be so depressing that they sap your energy.

Treat yourself in a calm, mature, self-respecting manner, just as you would treat any guest — or even a stranger — in your home. You deserve such treatment, and the self-esteem it engenders. Agree to that, won't you?

What have you done right today? You saw that if you treat yourself as a naughty child, constantly upbraiding yourself, you devalue yourself.

Today's Action Plan: I will treat myself as an adult. I will not punish myself for mistakes, but begin again.

You Are Unique

Every individual has a place to fill in the world, and is
important in some respect, whether he chooses to be so
or not.

Nathaniel Hawthorne

MindStep number one is first because with an unshaka-
ble sense of your unique worth you can take charge of
your life. If you really believe that you are unique and
have an independent worth, you'll be a winner. When
things get tough, it is your absolute belief in your worth
that keeps you in Action. Do you understand that?

You are unique. In all history there has never been
another exactly like you. Think of it, eighty-two billion
people have lived on this earth, and you are one of a
kind. Furthermore, in all the next six billion years that
science tells us our sun will burn, there will never be
another you.

Don't miss the point. Uniqueness is not a guarantee of
success, whether it's in losing weight or anything else,
but it affirms that you can do for yourself what no one
else can do.

You are unlimited. Never send negative I-grams to
yourself: "I can't do that," "I always fail," or "I'm just
like my Uncle Fred, the slob." Never affirm self-limita-
tion. Affirm what you want to be. What you believe is
what you are. Say it, won't you?

What have you done right today? You have faced the
wonderful fact of your uniqueness and seen what its
affirmation can mean in your life. That's a lot to learn in
one day.

Today's Action Plan: I will continue to develop a solid
understanding of my unique worth. I will not limit, but
affirm myself.

December 21

Always Be on Your Side

Happiness has many roots, but none more important
than security.

E. R. Stettinius, Jr.

Do you feel the need for some breathing space? If so, you're scheduling too much into a day. There are things you must do and there are things that can wait, giving you some necessary openness in your day. You can also feel crowded when friends or family members try to fill your empty moments with their own priorities. Don't always let them. It's important to have spaces in your day, isn't it?

Do you ever feel that you have little control over the direction of your day? It may sound a bit silly, but a way to feel in control is to rearrange something. It can be as simple as straightening a cupboard or desk drawer, or as major as emptying your appointment book for a day. Juggling your routine to make it work better for you helps you feel in control and secure. It's important to your new LifeWay to have a feeling of power, a feeling that you can achieve what you are working for.

Being on your own side is simply a way to express self-consideration. You need that attitude to become a winner. It's nice to have a considerate ally, like yourself, isn't it? Say YES.

What have you done right today? You took your own side. Whether you needed relaxing, empty spaces in your day, or a sense that you are master of your own direction, you took the necessary steps.

Today's Action Plan: I will set priorities to include some empty space. I will arrange schedules that work best for me.

December 22

The Overdoer

Untangling problems takes purpose, patience,
and persistence.

Frank Tyger

In most of this book, we dealt with the need for an overeater to get into Action. But there's another kind of overeater, in the minority to be sure, but with the opposite problem. This overeater is an overdoer, run ragged by a super-full schedule and the sense that the whole world rests on his or her shoulders. Do you know someone like that?

To overdoers, every activity is a "should." If they don't do it, it won't get done. Usually, this kind of overeater is really saying, "Don't look at my body, look at all the wonderful things I do." This attitude comes from a desperate need to be admired. But how can such people be admired without killing themselves in the process?

Try to choose between the tasks you love and the extras that are "shoulds." Begin to eliminate some of your work load, even though others admire how well you perform. This is tough, but you'll gain more time to devote to the jobs you decide to keep.

Learn to admire yourself for your true value, not just as a workhorse. Don't take on so much work that you are able to avoid the responsibility for your overeating. Then you'll be a natural for becoming a thinner-winner. That's true, isn't it?

What have you done right today? You saw that overdoing is another way to avoid responsibility for your overeating.

Today's Action Plan: I will concentrate on certain important jobs and let the rest go. I will act on my belief that my primary responsibility is to control my overeating.

356

Your Healing Mind

Undeniable evidence is emerging that the human mind can be trained to play an important part both in preventing disease and in overcoming it when it occurs.
Norman Cousins

The influence of mind on body was well known to ancient healers. However, scientific medicine focuses mostly on physical causes of illness. This is especially true for overweight. Fat is considered a disease of eating too much, and the cure is a reducing diet. Since diet alone has had little permanent effect on overweight, some doctors are coming to the conclusion that diet is only part of the answer. That makes sense, doesn't it?

Overeating can be influenced positively or negatively by your mental state. In other words, an event itself doesn't make you eat; it's how you react to it. For example, automobile trouble can send you to the refrigerator, or your tool chest, or the repair shop.

The brain doesn't eliminate old thinking habits. It simply overrides them by introducing new habits that compete with and finally replace the old. If you formerly gave yourself failure I-grams, now give some positive ones. If you used to be out of control, you now use self-management strategies that overwhelm the old helpless feelings. You know that if you put right-eating, exercise, and MindStep attitudes into your day, you will succeed. It's that simple, isn't it?

What have you done right today? You created attitudes of self-worth and control. You see that strong positive attitudes don't waste time dueling with old negative mindsets, they overcome them.

Today's Action Plan: I will follow a healing path. I will take good care of my mental state so my mind will take care of my body.

You Are Responsible

By the streets of "by and by," one arrives at the house of "never."
Saavedra M. de Cervantes

There is never a better time than today to build your own workable, comfortable, supremely livable LifeWay. If you are waiting for just the right time, you'll wait forever. You see that, don't you?

All people are responsible for their own happiness. If you have a scapegoat for your overeating ("Dad always made me clean my plate") you may be momentarily comforted, but it's a millstone, too. If you carry a grudge against someone ("If she loved me enough, I wouldn't overeat"), it makes only you miserable, no one else.

The only life you can control is your own, and then only one day at a time. Today is the only day you have to bring about meaningful changes in your life — not some future day.

You must be willing today to make the effort. You may have been living a right-eating, energized, positive, MindStep life for months, you may have had a significant weight loss — but you must be eager to make the effort today. Every day you need to make an intelligent and mature decision, and exchange the immediate gratification of overeating for a long-range, life-changing goal.

The question today and every day is: am I willing to do what it takes? The answer is YES.

What have you done right today? You accepted full responsibility for your life. You said YES to maturity.

Today's Action Plan: I will make a life-saving decision to take charge of my recovery. I will be eagerly responsible for all that I do today.

December 25

Peace Is Near

*All over the world people are seeking peace of mind, but
there can be no peace of mind
without strength of mind.*

Eric B. Gutkind

For almost a year you have been working on your
mental fitness, exercising your mind's muscles. Today
you are stronger than ever. There was a reason for this
emphasis on strength of mind. That reason was to have
you, through your own effort, declare peace within
yourself. Once you were in conflict, it seemed, with the
very air you breathed! The imbalance between what you
wanted (to stop overeating) and what you were actually
doing (overeating) created an unbearable disharmony.
Your life was a series of discordant notes. You needed
peace in your life, didn't you?

When you do what you know you need to do, peace
of mind envelops you like water surrounds the fish in it.
Peace, not food, becomes your element. You allow
nothing and no one to disturb this peace.

Above all you keep your mind in a state of calm. The
real destroyer of peace was always your own negative
thoughts. You have now learned to let go of distrust,
fear, and self-blame. You have willed your negative self-
critic to be silent and have filled your mind to the brim
with joy and peace.

You are truly in charge of your peace. Keep it with
you always, won't you?

What have you done right today? You saw clearly
that you were your own peacemaker. You are the
creative decision-maker of your life. You are the director
of your energy.

Today's Action Plan: I will make my mind strong so
that I can establish peace within myself. I will believe
that peace of mind comes through Action, that peace is
active, not passive.

December 26

Beating the Fear of Expectation

*I was not prepared to be thin. I was like the poor girl
who suddenly gets rich. How was I supposed to act?*
A Take Off Pounds Sensibly (TOPS) Queen

Reaching your natural weight, the one most comfortable
for you, is a moment of supreme joy, one of the happiest
in your life, and it should be. It took incredible courage
and persistence. Enjoy your new life. Walk through the
doors now open to you. Be prepared for the success you
deserve, won't you?

When you began your program, you went through a
transformation. It was exciting and people praised you
along the way. But your new body and attitudes are
now a fact. You are no longer The Dieter, who needs
special consideration. This is the time when you are
expected to perform at home, on the job, and at social
occasions.

Sometimes when we reach our natural weight, we fear
the expectations of others. We ask, "What do they want
of me?"

People may say, "You look wonderful. You don't need
to take all these precautions any more." Don't you
believe it! You must keep doing all those things that got
you to this day. Carry on with your good eating
management to stabilize and maintain your weight.
Continue your physical fitness routine. Practice the
Action MindStep principles; they're the bedrock of your
new LifeWay. Persevere and stay healthy, won't you?

What have you done right today? You saw that the
way to whip the fear of expectation is to continue all
those things that made you a thinner winner.

**Today's Action Plan: I will take charge of weight
stabilization. I will continue to use Action MindStep
attitudes.**

Diet without Exercise Is No Diet at All

The bathroom scale tells you you're doing something
right, but you actually haven't improved
your body composition.

Donald Layman

The nutritionist quoted above conducted an interesting experiment on a group of obese rats. They starved off 75 percent of their body weight, yet maintained the same proportion of fat. In other words, these rats went from being big and fat to being small and fat. And worse, if they regained their weight, the proportion of body fat increased even more. The same thing applies to people who diet but don't exercise. Paradoxically, the former dieters end up fatter for having dieted. That's the last straw, isn't it?

The answer lies in right-eating plus exercise. On this kind of schedule, your energized body gets into the habit of burning off fat. When you reach your maintenance weight, you may actually need to eat more just to keep your weight from going too low!

It's too bad exercise isn't called play-ercise. Perhaps fewer overweights would have trouble with the idea. Think of it. Fat disappearing while you play! Isn't that a wonderful mental image? Now that you've thought about it, do it.

You'll begin to love your play-ercise game. Just keep a happy balance between food intake and energy outgo. To win, all you need is the commitment. Isn't that right?

What have you done right today? You were reminded that diet with exercise is a winning proposition. You committed yourself to Action on every front.

Today's Action Plan: I will think of exercise as the game that destroys fat forever. I will put myself in control of my life and never let go.

What Would You Wish?

For of all sad words of tongue or pen
The saddest are these: "It might have been!"
John Greenleaf Whittier

Right now, do you have everything you want from life? Not many people do, but we certainly feel happier when we're heading in the right direction. Are you headed right?

Many people who have lived a full life span don't so much regret what they have done as what they haven't done. Pretend you are eighty and lamenting your failure to do a certain thing. Which experience do you regret missing? Did overweight, either in a real or imagined way, prevent you from achieving your desire?

Pretend:

> • It might have been that, had you worked for achievement, the work after awhile would have taken on a rhythm. What looked impossible would have happened.
> • It might have been that you constantly lamented the fact that life was not fair. Life might have been good and joyous, but you did not rescue the joy from the trap of emotional pain.
> • It might have been that life gave you a chance to be what you could have been, experience what you could have experienced, and love what you could have loved.

Some day will you look back and say sadly, "It might have been"? Or will you say with satisfaction, "It was"? It's your choice, isn't it?

What have you done right today? You determined that you will experience all today has to offer.

Today's Action Plan: I will work to realize my ambition. I will not take refuge from problems in overeating, but in Action MindStep principles.

December 29

What Do You Have to Live for?

I believe that only one person in a thousand knows the trick of really living in the present.

Storm Jameson

Every minute of the day is an unrepeatable miracle for us to use. Let's use these small miracles to strengthen our attitudes toward ourselves and our place in the world. Our minds are fortresses, impenetrable by good or bad. Only we can choose to surrender, fight, or survive. You have a strong sense of survial. Use it each minute, won't you?

Today is yours for Action and imagination. Taking charge of your life is an act of imagination. It is a search through your desires, a lifelong discovery process.

Have you noticed in time-lapse photography how a rose gradually diplays its inner self? One petal at a time unfolds until it has created its own full-blown, open-hearted beauty. Each minute of today is like a rose petal. As your day unfolds, you create a harmonious, beautiful LifeWay, free forever of the pain of overeating. By tonight you will be in full bloom, won't you?

What have you done right today? You used every minute of today to take practical Action for weight control, and to search for the desires that power your determination.

Today's Action Plan: I will bloom, using the Action process of living in the present. I will give myself all the time I need to discover the beauty within me.

Think of Yourself as a Winner

*Have you learned lessons only of those who admired
you, and were tender with you, and stood aside for you?
Have you not learned great lessons from those who
rejected you, and braced themselves against you, or
disputed the passage with you?*

Walt Whitman

We've all stumbled at times. But here you are on this
special day, marching ahead, risking and learning —
even from those who don't accept you. Such courage as
yours is the basis of security, self-value, and ability to
achieve. Your courage defeats any dependency on overeating. You have grown up. You are an adult who
refuses to be handicapped by a food pacifier. That's true,
isn't it?

• Think of yourself as a winner today when
you function in a crisis without overeating.
• Think of yourself as a winner when you
truly believe that people love and value you
just as you are — and you do, too.
• Think of yourself as a winner when you
risk your feelings to accomplish what you
know needs to be done.
• Think of yourself as a winner when you
refuse to retreat from your problems in food.
• Think of yourself as a winner when you
practice your new LifeWay. Think of yourself that way, won't you?

What have you done right today? You learned from
others, but you got your sense of meaning from within.
You have a purpose and goals.

Today's Action Plan: I will think of myself as an
independent adult who no longer needs a food pacifier. I
will think of myself as a winner.

December 31

More Can Be Grasped

Not the whole [of life], oh, of course, not the whole . . .
but much more than you might suppose.
Keep going, don't quit. Imagine. Scrutinize.
Once more with feeling: think.

James McConkey

There is no last word to this book. The story doesn't
end; it just keeps beginning again. But each time it
begins, each time you plant positive thoughts in your
mind or take charge of your eating, you become much
more independent, a lot more effective. How complex
you are, and how wonderful! You deserve to grasp so
much more of life. Please agree, won't you?

Some days it seems as if your positive thoughts refuse
to take root. Believe that they will. Change is hard, but
you can do it. Change is the root of all achievement.

Together we have come to the end of your beginning.
Many messages have been sent to you through these
pages. Perhaps some were not received. But as the
Japanese philosopher Segaki said, "Just because the message may not be received never means it is not worth
sending." Next year, as you dip into these pages again,
there will be new messages waiting here for you.

It has been a long journey, but one well worth taking.
That's true, isn't it? Say YES.

What have you done right today? As always, you
have renewed your commitment to right-eating and
physical and mental fitness. You have made the Twelve
Action MindSteps the focus of your new LifeWay. You
have made yourself a winner.

Today's Action Plan: I will realize that today is as
much of a challenge and opportunity as the first day of
the year. I will commit myself anew to uncovering my
essential self.

About the Author

Jeane Westin is the author of six books, including *The Thin Book* and *Break Out of Your Fat Cell*, both from CompCare Publishers. Her books have been selected by book clubs and reprinted by magazines.

More than 250 of her articles have appeared in national publications such as *Ms.*, *Woman's Day*, *Parade*, *Weight Watchers*, and many others.

She has taught writing at American River College and has been a featured speaker for writers' organizations, colleges, and professional groups. Jeane has been interviewed on many television and radio programs, including "Donahue," "Good Morning, America," and "The Today Show."

Jeane Westin is a member of the Authors Guild and is listed in *Who's Who of American Women* and *Working Press of the Nation*. She has been honored for her literary achievements by the Sacramento Regional Arts Council. She is a lifetime honorary member of the California Writers Club.

Subject Index

Subject Index

Subject Index